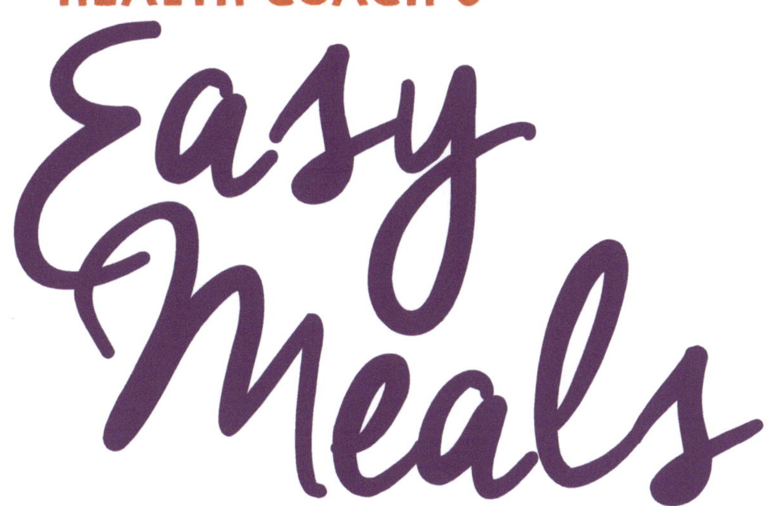

Sonia Bhatia, MBA, INHC
www.beinghealthylivingwell.com
beinghealthylivingwell@gmail.com

Amy Pabbi, MS. INHC. RHC
www.Amarwellnessinc.com
Amarwellnessinc@gmail.com

Ordering Information: Quantity sales. Special discounts are available on quantity purchases by corporations, associations, and others. For details, contact the publisher at the address above.

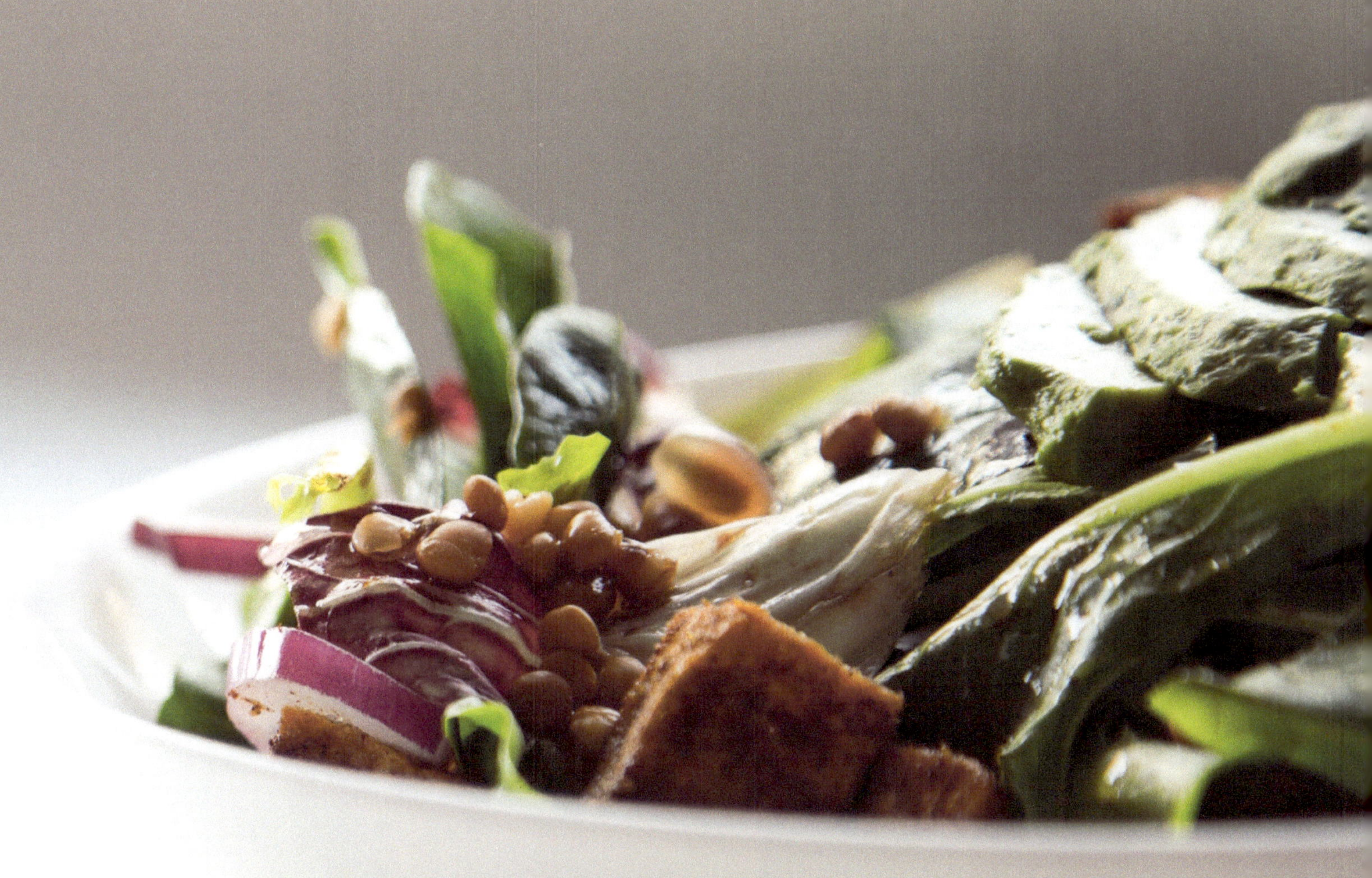

HEALTH COACH'S
Easy
Meals
VEGETARIAN / GLUTEN FREE

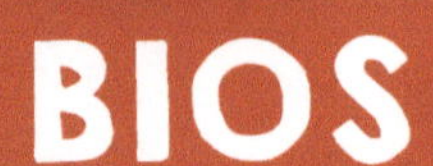

BIOS

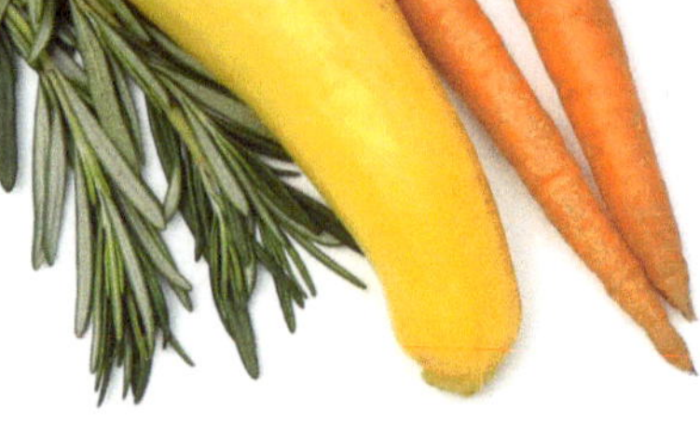

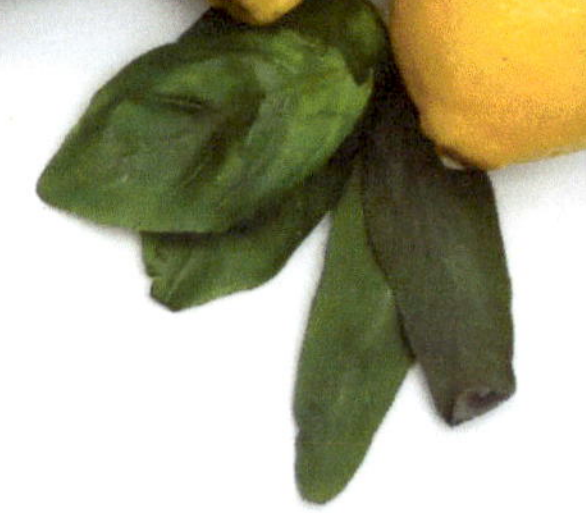

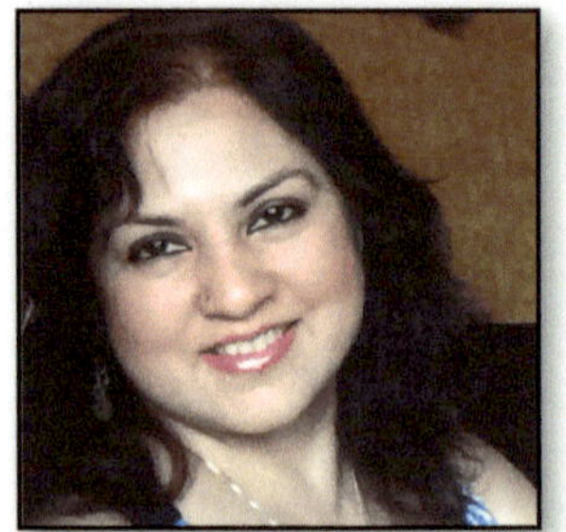

Sonia Bhatia, MBA, INHC

"I am a Certified Integrative Nutrition Health Coach. I focus on overall health and wellness through diet, nutrition and lifestyle transformation. My approach is holistic and emphasizes long-term sustainability. As a health coach I will work with you to reach your health goals in areas such as achieving optimal weight, reducing food cravings, increasing and improving sleep, and maximizing your energy. As your partner I will help you develop a deeper understanding of the food and lifestyle choices that work best for you and implement lasting changes that will improve your energy, balance, and health".

Sonia is trained and certified by The Institute for Integrative Nutrition in New York and Board approved by The American Association on Drug-less Practitioners.

She is passionate about health and wellness. She is a home chef and enjoys traveling to explore new cultures and culinary feats!

www.beinghealthylivingwell.com   beinghealthylivingwell@gmail.com

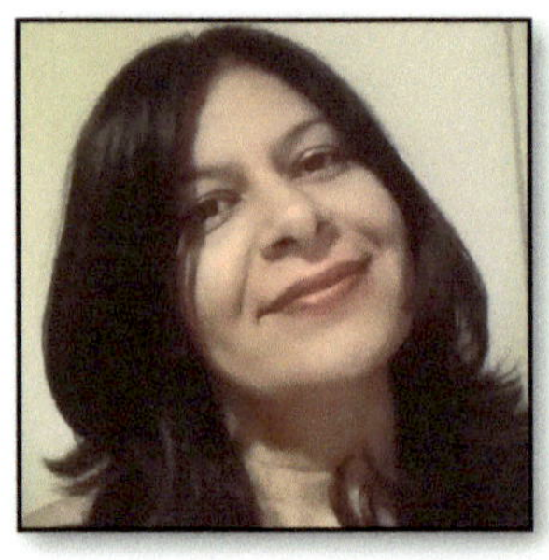

Amy Pabbi, MS. INHC. RHC

Amy Pabbi is a board certified health coach who supports people in learning how to how to optimize their diets with her knowledge of nutrition". She received her MS in Nutrition and training as integrated health coach from IIN (Institute of Integrated Nutrition). Using her extensive knowledge she helps clients feel great by uncovering hidden food intolerances and helping them transfer to a healthy lifestyle.

Amy lives with her husband and two lovely teenaged kids and her two dogs Aslan and Bruno. She was born and raised in India and moved in Canada in 2004 where she quickly learned that the Indian community was developing a stronger appetite towards fast and processed foods rather than their traditional culture of cooking food at home. It's not easy to resettle in a new country. Being in immigrant she understands how stressful it is to take care of kids, job, managing work and life balance. She knows when you are new to the country you think all the colorful foods on shelf looks healthy. But no one knows the ugly truth in those sugar coated food items. She realized that as a result of a convenient lifestyle people are getting generally unhealthier and are not aware that food has a big role in their health.

Amy would like to remind and educate her community that going back to the basics is the mantra of healthy living. This book is the materialization of her efforts to reintroduce Indian cooking in a new, healthier way. This book is just not for someone who likes Indian food but for everyone who is looking for healthy cooking with Indian flavor.

www.Amarwellnessinc.com   Amarwellnessinc@gmail.com

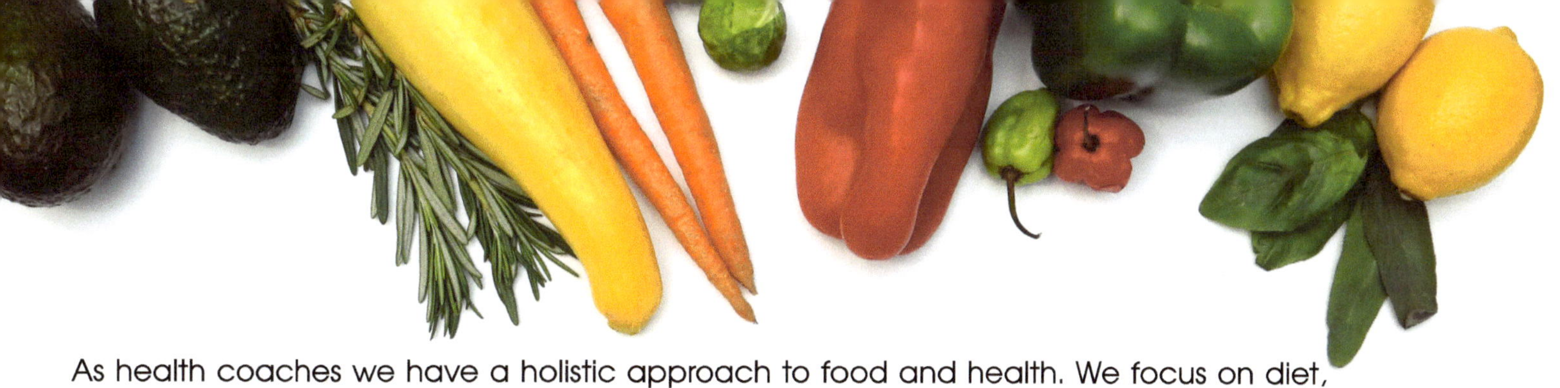

As health coaches we have a holistic approach to food and health. We focus on diet, nutrition and overall wellness by focusing on consuming nutrient dense and unprocessed whole foods. Based on our training, knowaledge and experience we have created recipes that are not only delicious and flavorful but provide the nutrition our body needs to function and thrive optimally. This compilation of our favorite 30 recipes is unique in that:

- Every ingredient used in the recipes adds nutrition in terms of macronutrients (lean protein, complex carbohydrates, heart healthy fats) and micronutrients (Vitamins and Minerals)
- Recipes are clean and unprocessed meaning they are whole foods and have not been processed in any manner to alter their nutrition value.
- Recipes do not include food groups such as dairy as research shows that it can cause inflammation in some people so we have substituted it with a healthy alternative such as Coconut Milk which adds heart healthy fats
- There is no processed sugar in any recipe. Natural sweeteners such as honey and fruits have been used to provide sweetness
- All recipes are vegetarian catering to anyone who follows a vegetarian diet or needs to add vegetables and fruits to their diet to benefit from the vitamins and minerals that fruits and vegetables bring such as:
  - Potassium and Magnesium and Vitamin E in Spinach
  - Zucchini contains Vitamin B6 and C and K along with Potassium and Manganese
  - Cauliflower which is a great source of Fiber and Vitamins C and K
  - Mango a delicious fruit with Vitamin C and Vitamin A
- Only the most nutrient dense oils have been used such as Extra Virgin Olive Oil, Coconut Oil and Ghee (clarified butter) so as to provide essential healthy fats and Omega 3s
- Ingredients used provide anti-inflammatory, Anti-bacterial properties e.g.: honey, ginger, garlic, turmeric and coconut oil
- Our recipes are Gluten Free – no wheat, barley or rye
- Herbs and spices have been used to not only add flavor and taste but to add nutrition and health healing benefits e.g.: Cilantro, Mint, Cinnamon, Ginger, Garlic
- Finally these recipes are light on the digestive system and Quick and Easy to cook not taking a lot of time to prep or create

We hope you will cook these recipes for these simple reasons:
- They are nutrient dense
- They are great for weight management
- They include natural and healing ingredients
- They are quick and easy
- And they come with love and warmth from our kitchen to yours !!

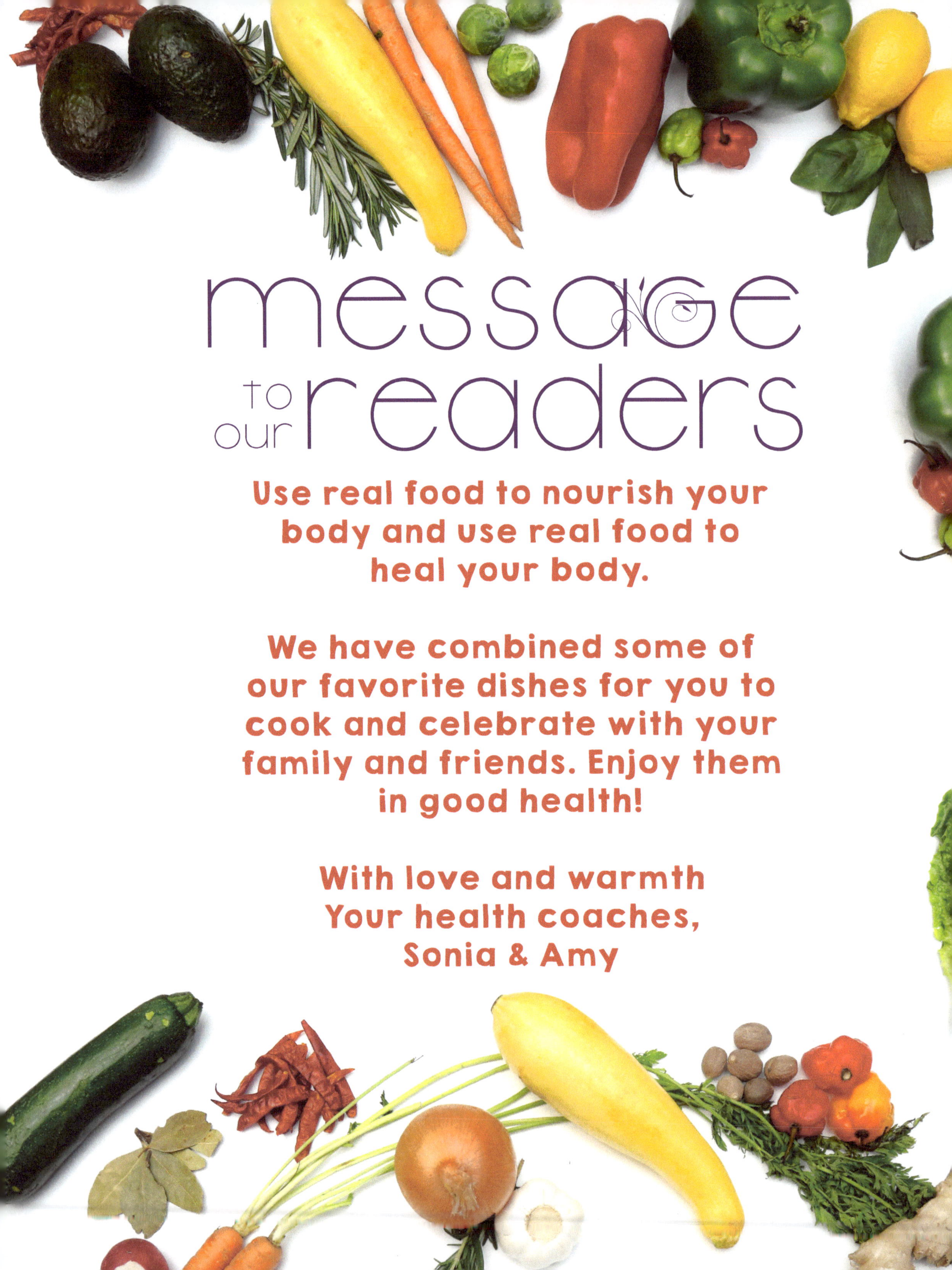

message
to our readers

Use real food to nourish your body and use real food to heal your body.

We have combined some of our favorite dishes for you to cook and celebrate with your family and friends. Enjoy them in good health!

With love and warmth
Your health coaches,
Sonia & Amy

TABLE OF CONTENTS

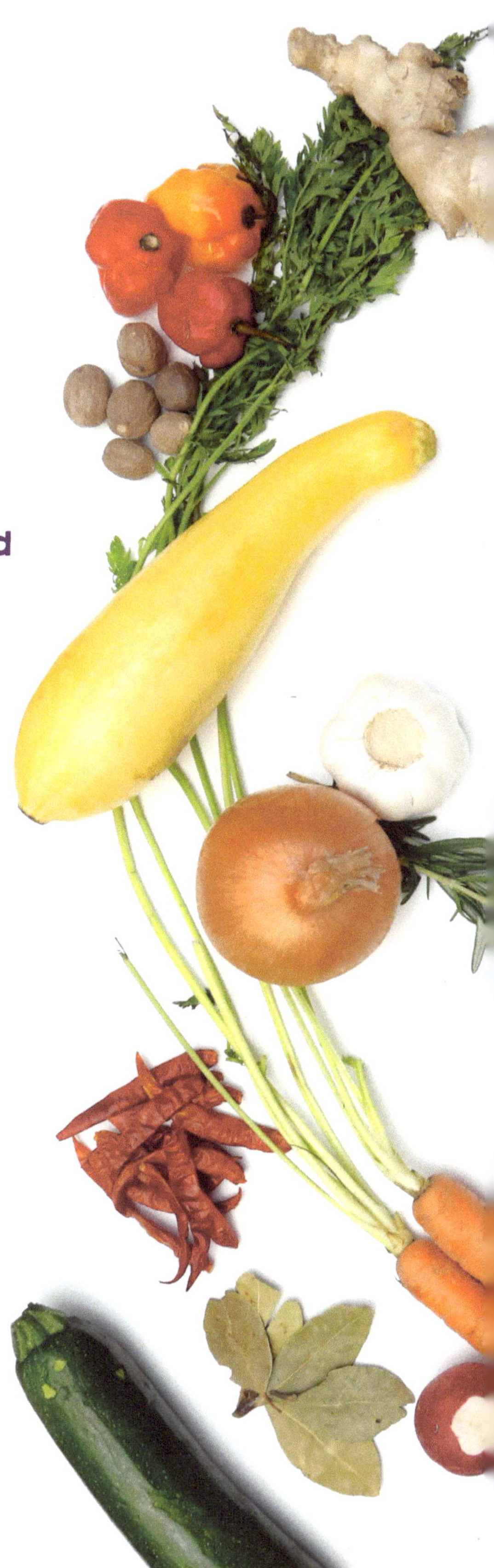

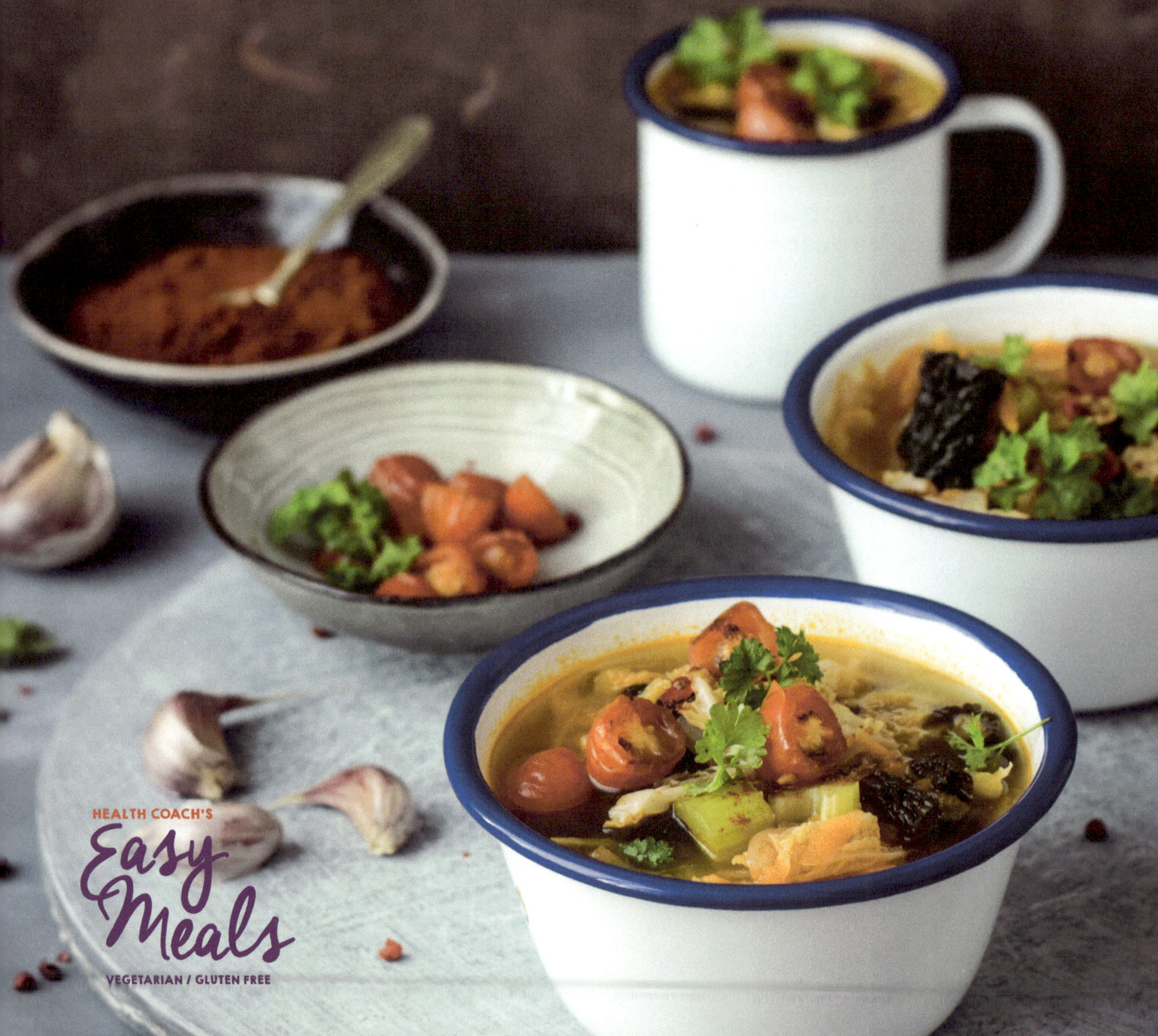

Nature is so smart it
put medicine in food

- David Wolfe

HEALTH COACH'S
Easy
Meals
VEGETARIAN / GLUTEN FREE

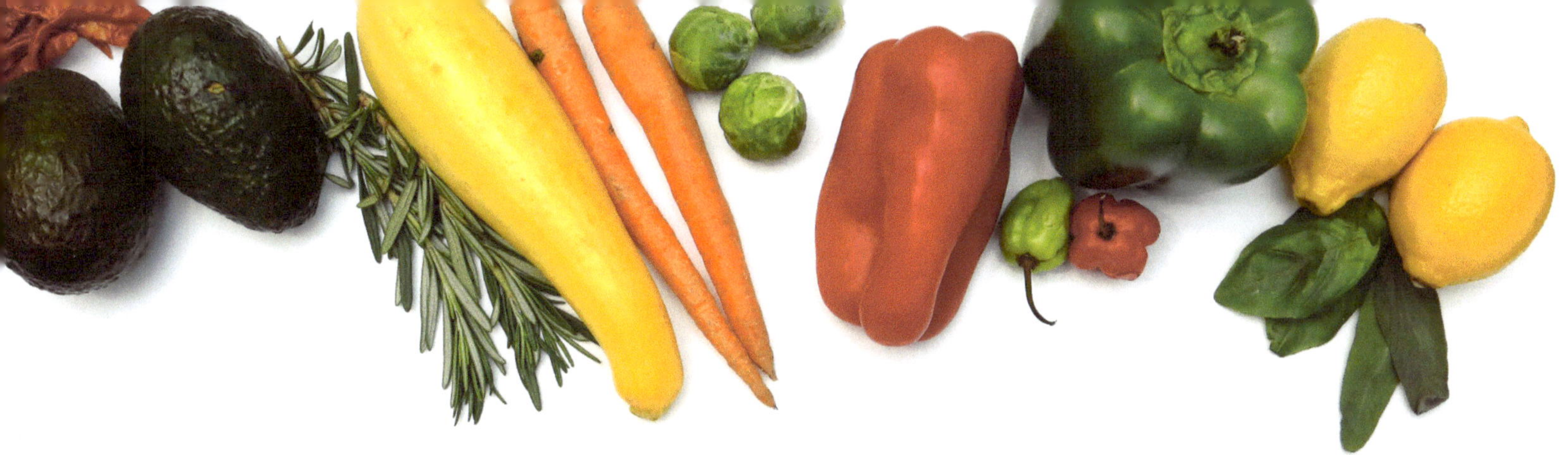

SOUPS

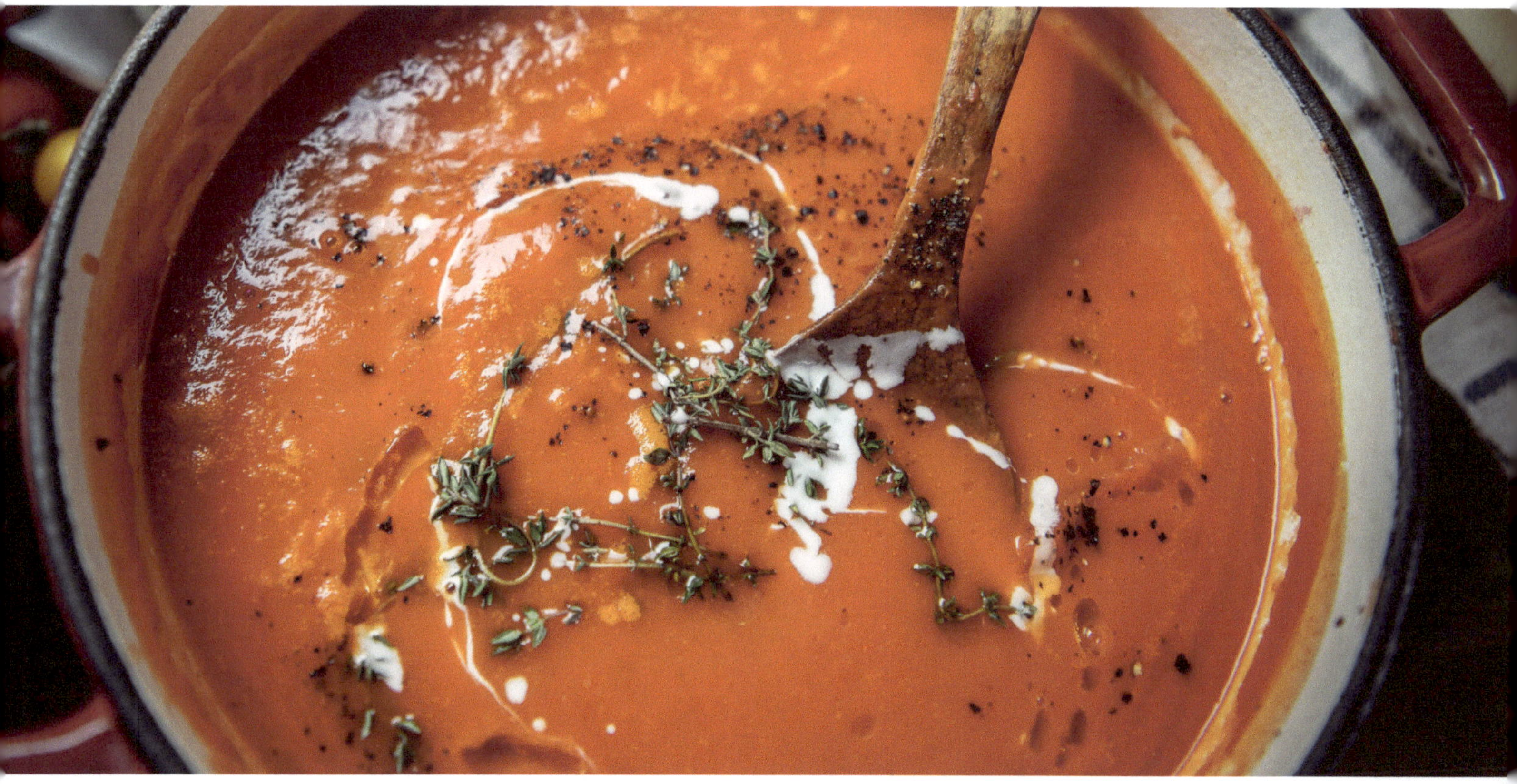

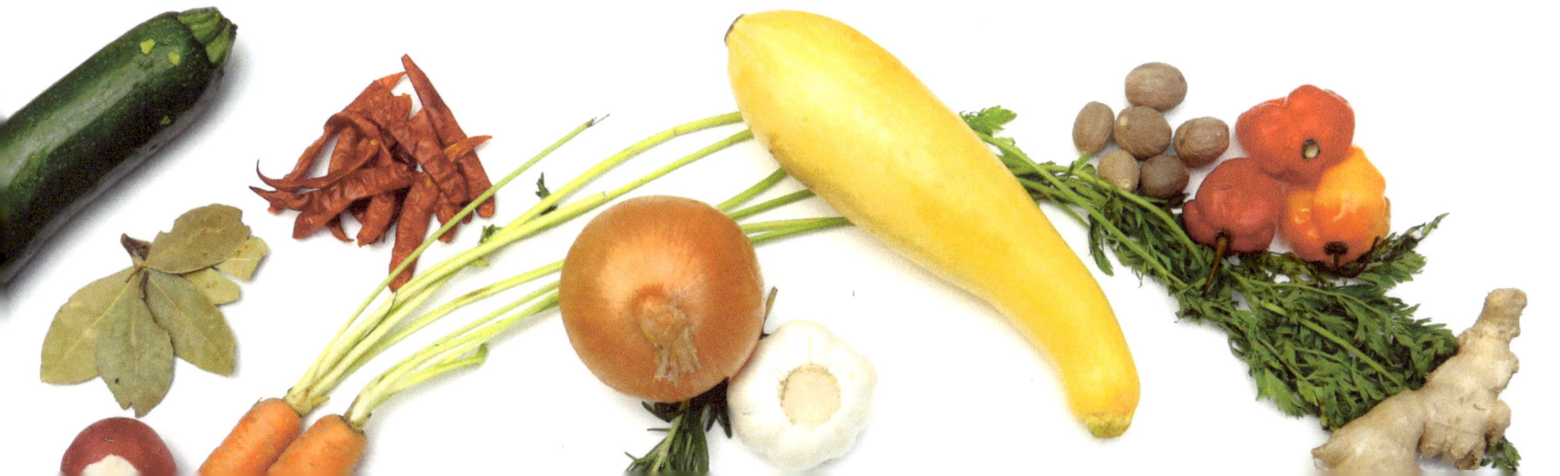

Tomato Basil Soup

INGREDIENTS

- 1 tablespoon extra-virgin olive oil
- 1 1/2 cups onion (chopped)
- 3 garlic cloves, minced
- 3/4 cup chopped fresh basil
- 1 (28-ounce) can fire-roasted diced tomatoes
- 1 cup full fat coconut milk
- 1/4 teaspoon salt
- 1/4 teaspoon black pepper

DIRECTIONS

1. Heat olive oil in a saucepan over medium-high heat.
2. Add onion; sauté 3 minutes.
3. Stir in garlic; cook for 1 minute.
4. Add basil and tomatoes; bring to a boil.
5. Place mixture in blender, and blend until smooth.
6. Return to pan; stir in coconut milk, salt, and pepper.
7. Return to medium-high; cook 2 minutes.
8. Serve topped with fresh basil!

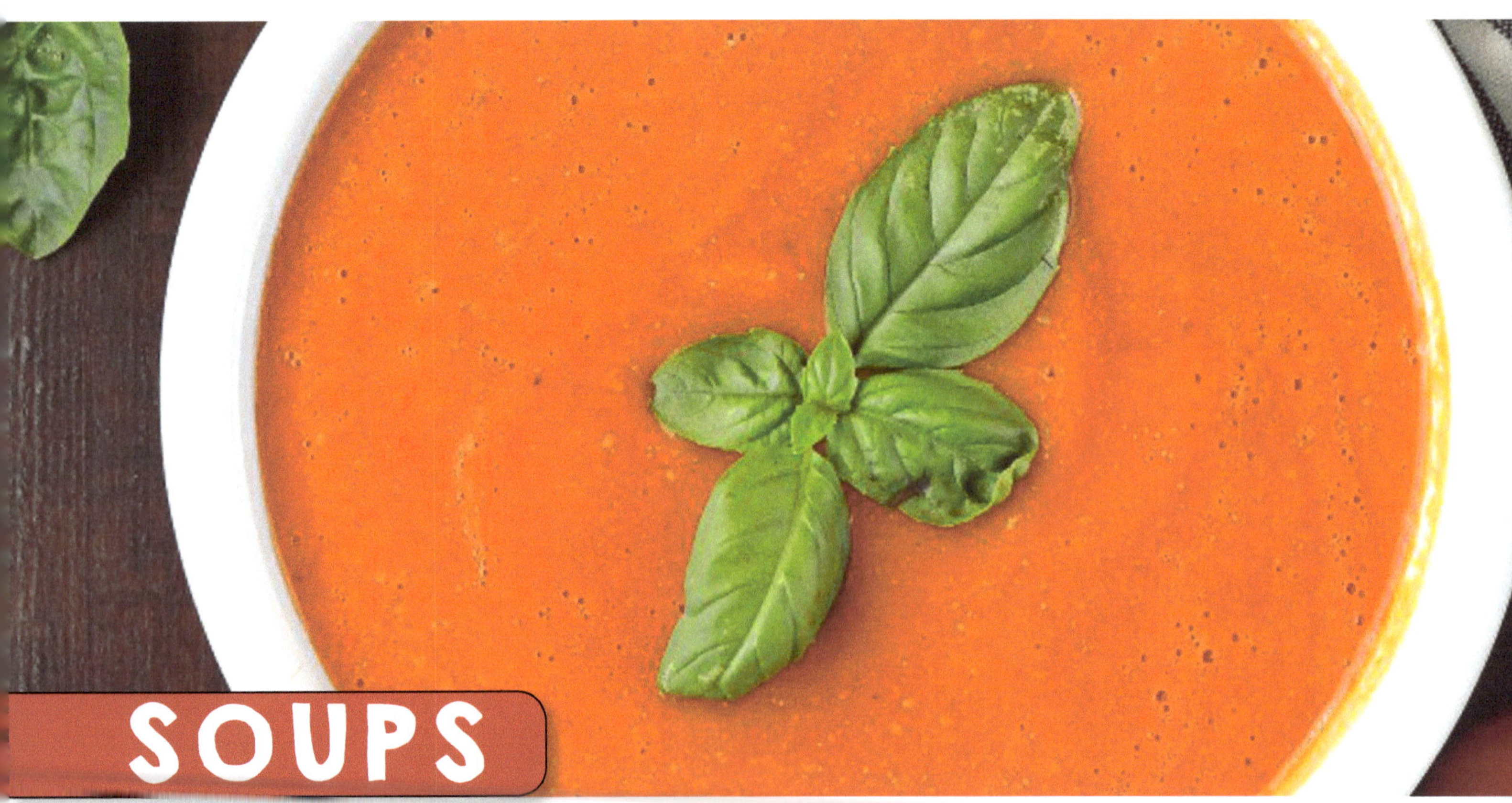

Cream of Spinach Soup

INGREDIENTS

- 2 cups (packed) spinach
- 1 onion, quartered;
- 2 cloves garlic, sliced;
- 4 cups vegetable stock
- 2 tbsp. coconut milk;
- 2 tablespoons olive oil or coconut oil
- Sea salt and freshly ground black pepper

DIRECTIONS

1. Melt oil in a saucepan placed over a medium heat.
2. Add the onion, garlic and spinach and cook for 4 to 5 minutes.
3. Add the vegetable stock, season to taste with salt and pepper, and bring to a boil.
4. Lower the heat, cover, and let simmer about 20 minutes.
5. Remove from the heat; add the coconut milk, and purée with an immersion blender (or pour into a standalone blender).
6. Adjust the seasoning and serve hot.

Mushroom Cauliflower Soup

INGREDIENTS

- 1 tbsp olive oil or coconut oil
- 1 yellow onion, chopped
- 2 cloves of fresh garlic, crushed
- ½ large head of cauliflower head , chopped coarsely
- 12 ounces of mushrooms chopped coarsely
- 2 ½-3 cups vegetable broth
- Sea salt and pepper, to taste

DIRECTIONS

1. Wash, prepare, chop and slice vegetables.
2. Heat oil in large pot and sauté over a low to medium heat until the onion and garlic are translucent.
3. Add in the cauliflower and mushrooms and stir for a few minutes.
4. Add the vegetable stock and season to taste and bring to a boil then turn down the heat and simmer for 15 minutes or until the vegetables are soft. Add more water/stock if needed.
5. Once cooked, blend the soup until smooth.

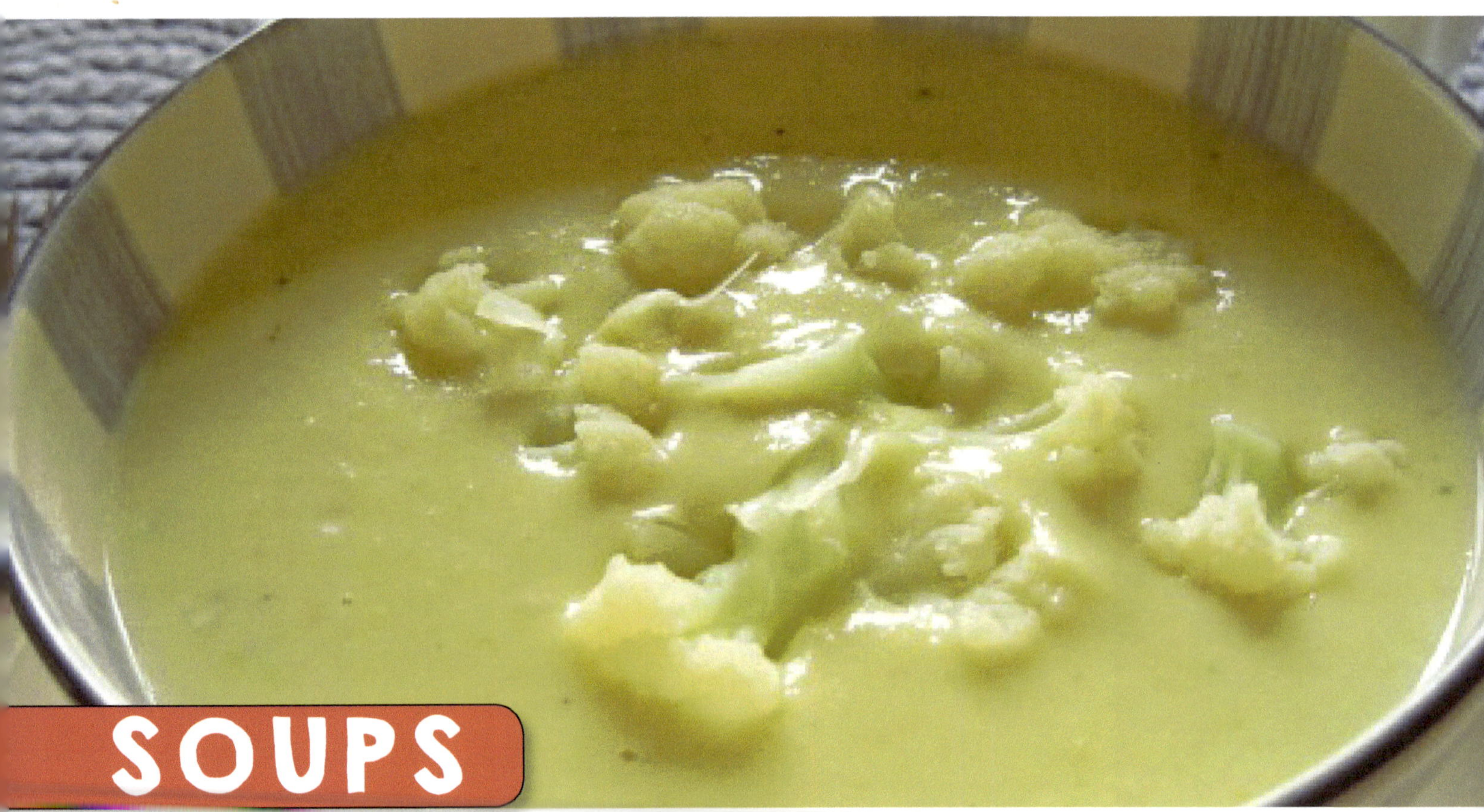

Lentil Soup

INGREDIENTS

- 1 1/2 cups red lentils
- 1 teaspoon turmeric
- 1/2 teaspoon cayenne pepper
- 1 teaspoon cumin
- 1/4 teaspoon cardamom
- 2 -3 curry leaves or 2 -3 bay leaves
- 6 cups vegetable stock
- 3 tablespoons clarified butter (ghee)
- 2 teaspoons mustard seeds
- 2 garlic cloves, finely chopped
- salt and pepper
- 1/2-1 lemon

DIRECTIONS

1. Rinse the lentils.
2. Bring to a boil with the stock, turmeric, Cayenne, cumin, cardamom and curry/bay leaves.
3. Let simmer until the lentils are very soft approx. 30 minutes
4. If using bay leaves, remove them now. Curry leaves can be left in the soup.
5. Run the soup quickly in a blender to a not too smooth consistency
   (or mash the lentils with a ladle).
6. Sautee the garlic and mustard seeds lightly in the fat and add to the soup.
7. Let simmer for another 5 minutes.
8. Add salt, pepper and squeezed lemon to taste.

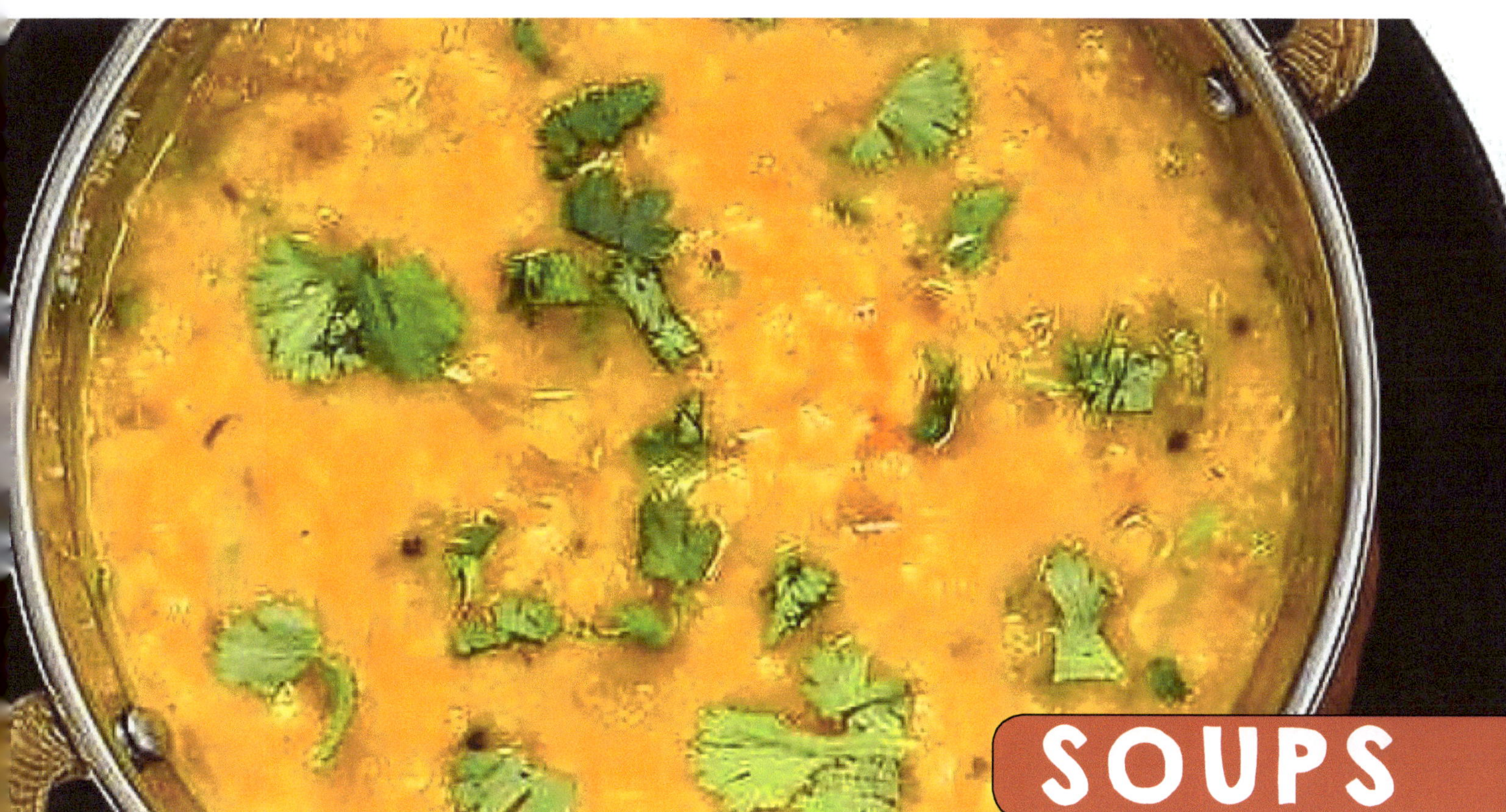

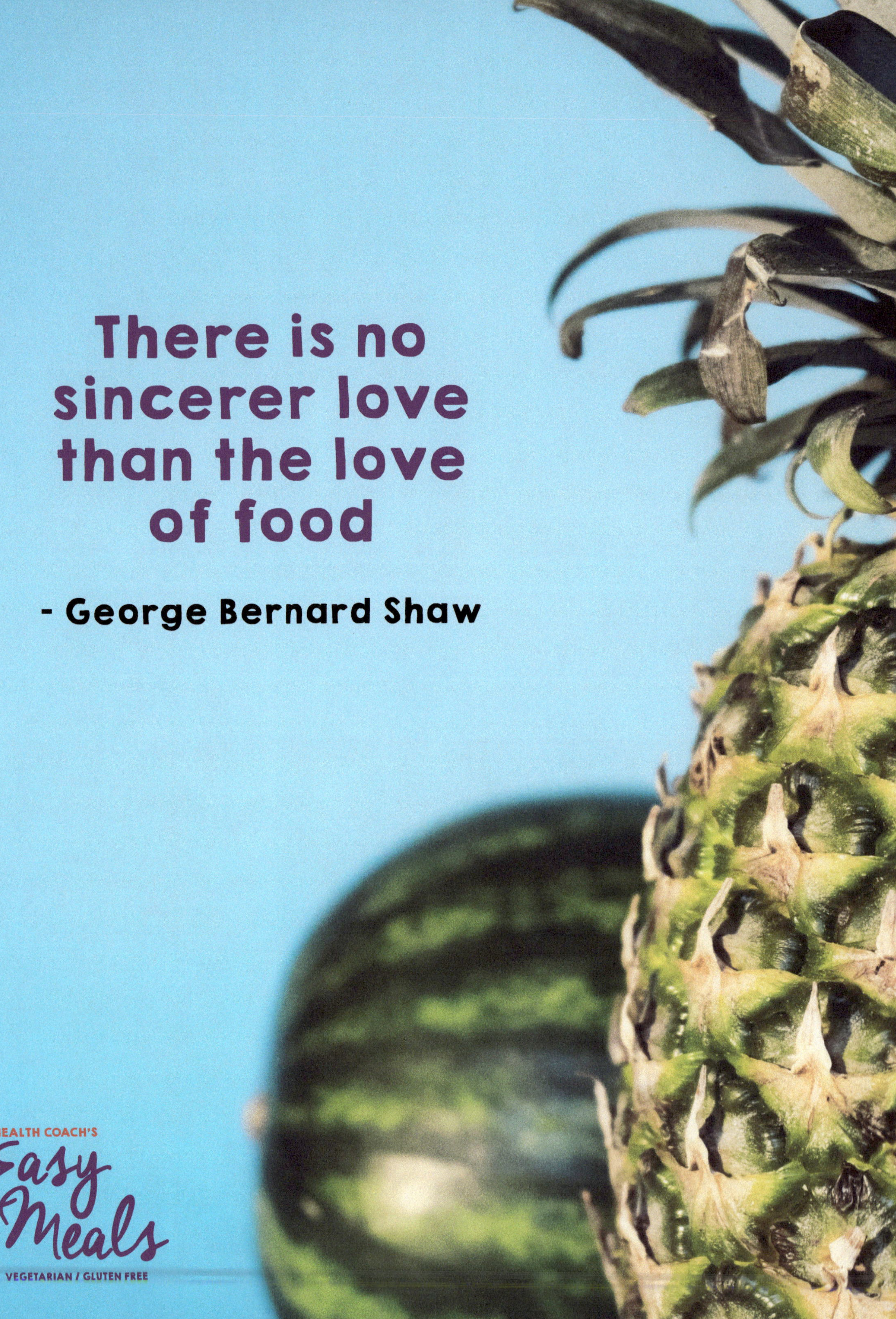

There is no sincerer love than the love of food

- George Bernard Shaw

HEALTH COACH'S
Easy Meals
VEGETARIAN / GLUTEN FREE

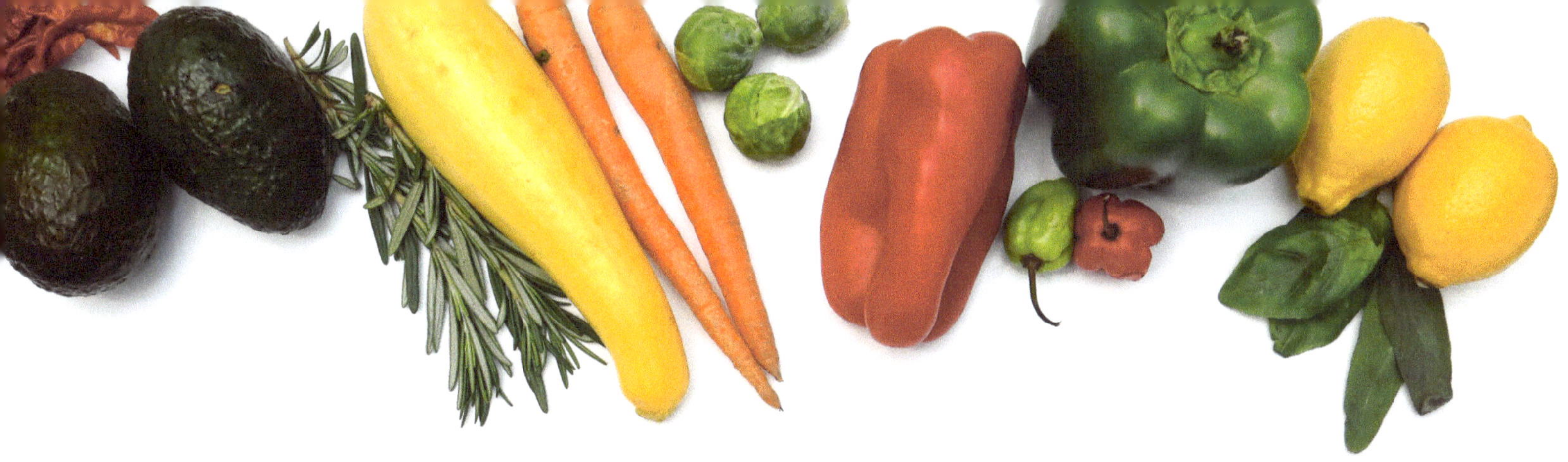

SNACKS

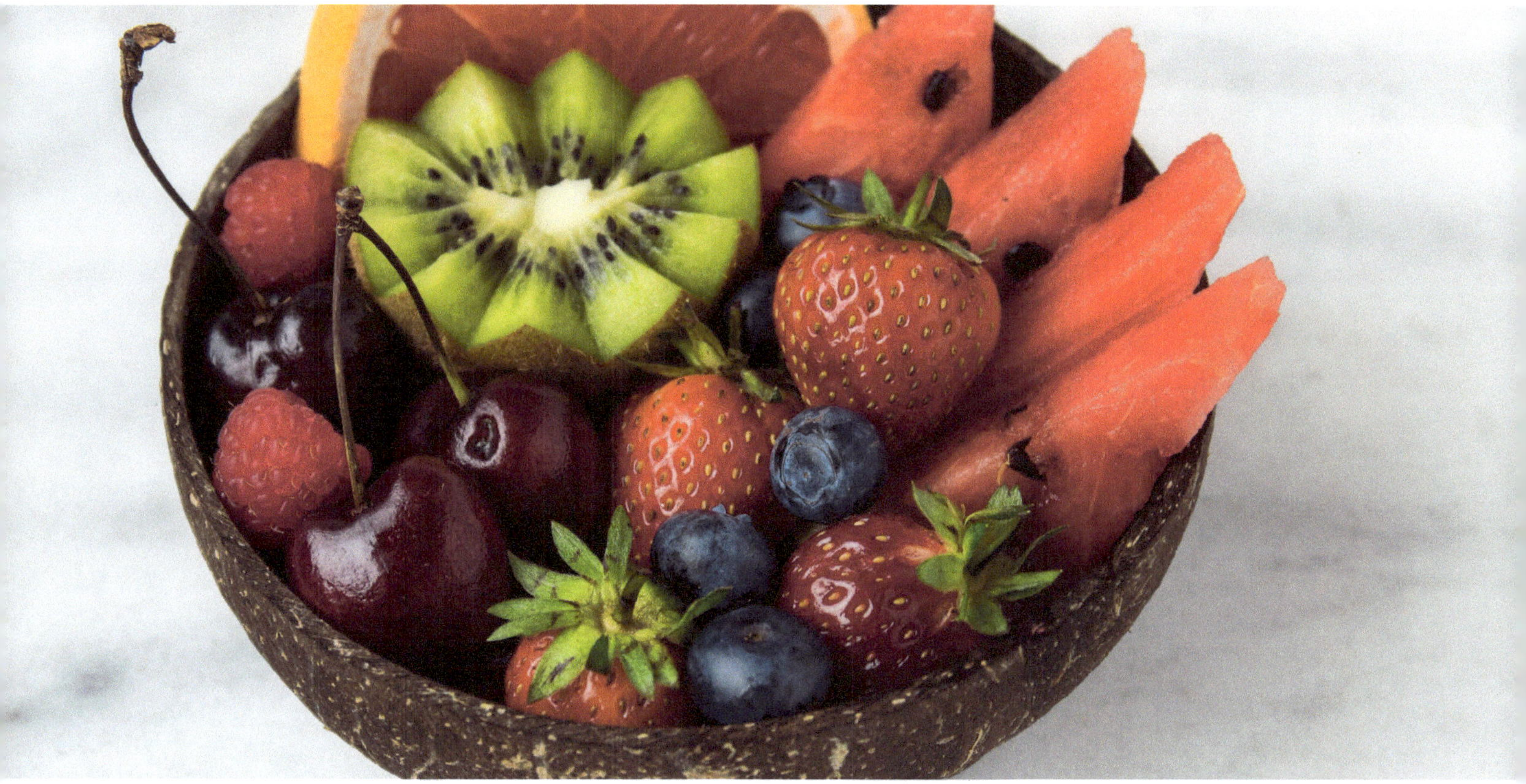

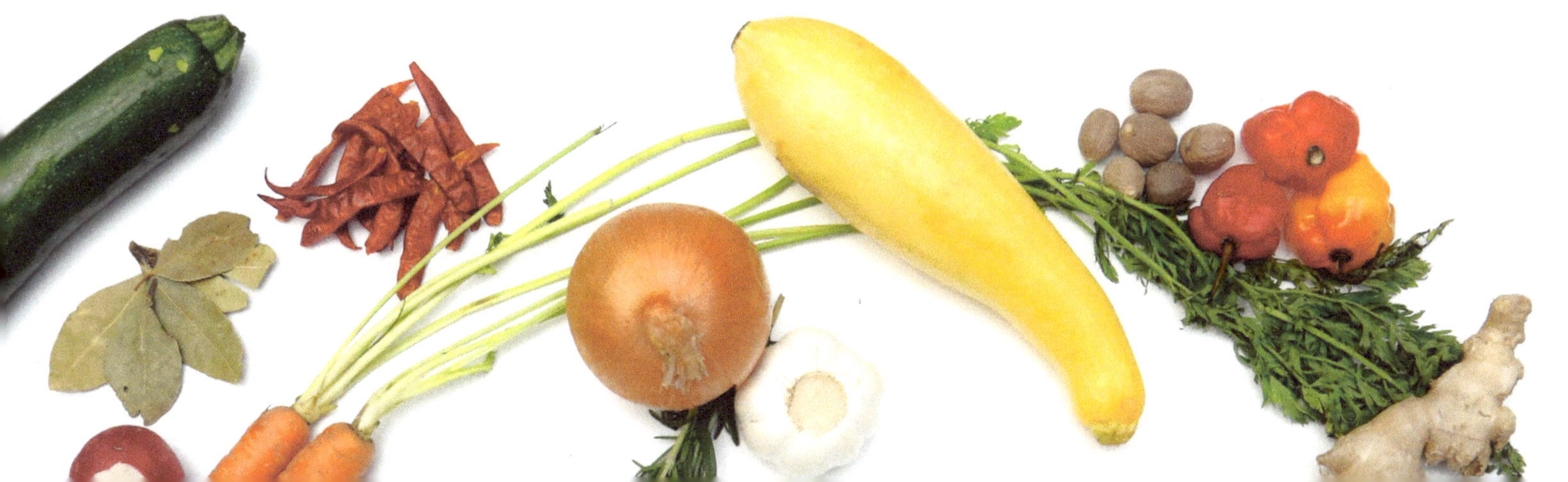

Basil Hummus

INGREDIENTS

- 1 15 oz can of chickpeas
- 1 garlic clove
- Juice of 1 lemon
- 1/4 cup tahini
- 2 cups packed basil leaves
- Salt and fresh cracked black pepper

DIRECTIONS

1. Drain and rinse the chickpeas. Put them in food processor along with the smashed garlic clove. Process the chickpeas for several minutes, stopping to scrape down the sides of the bowl as necessary. Process the beans first to get them as smooth as possible.
2. Add the tahini and lemon to the puree and process briefly to combine. Then add the basil, and process for another couple of minutes, scraping down the sides as needed.
3. Season with salt and fresh cracked black pepper.

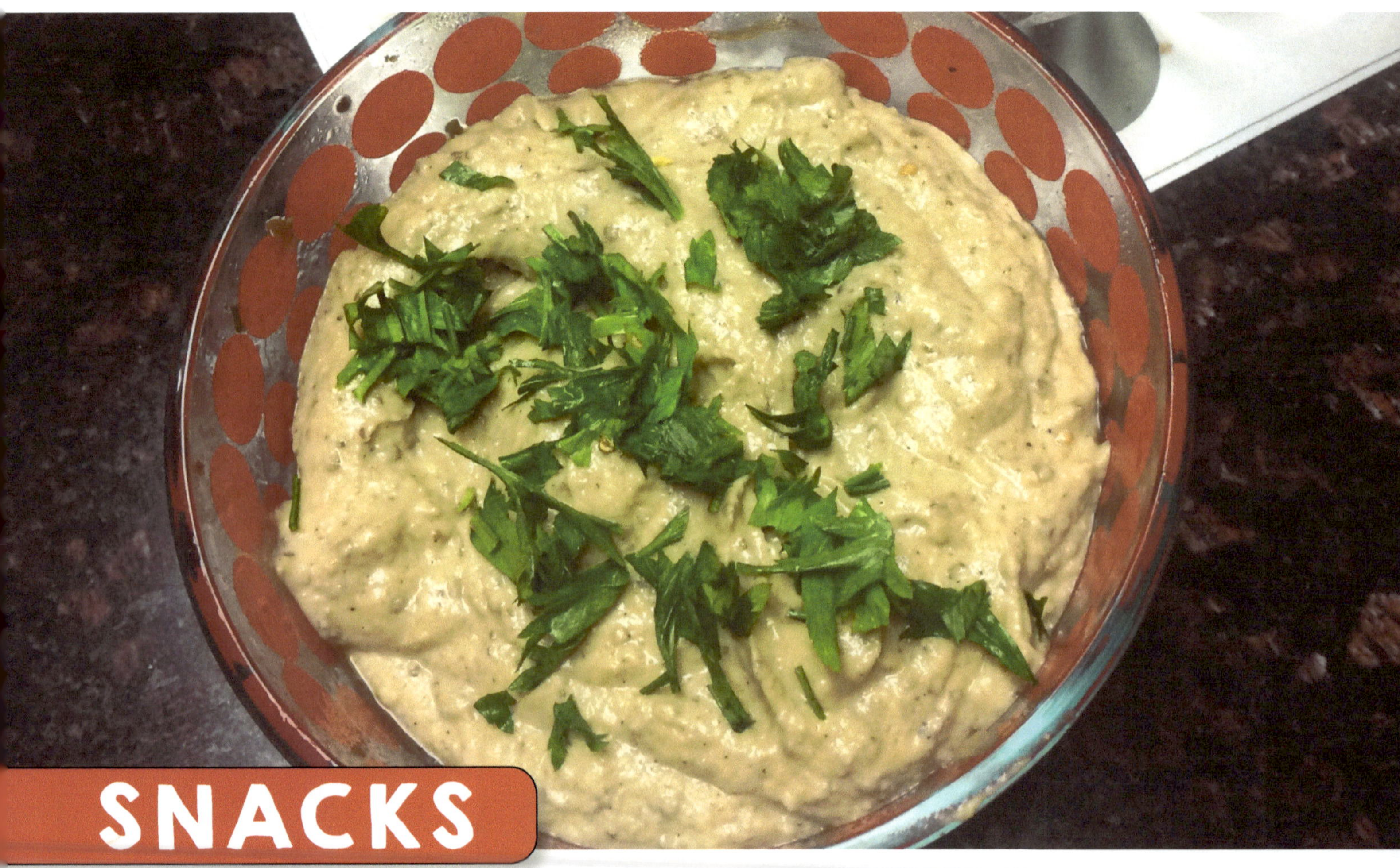

SNACKS

Granola

INGREDIENTS

- 1 cup raw walnuts, chopped
- 1 cup dried apples, chopped (or another choice of nuts like cashews)
- 1 cup dried cranberries
- 1 cup raw sunflower seeds
- ½ cup raw almonds, chopped
- Pinch of ground clove, cinnamon and nutmeg

DIRECTIONS

1. Combine all ingredients in a bowl and serve

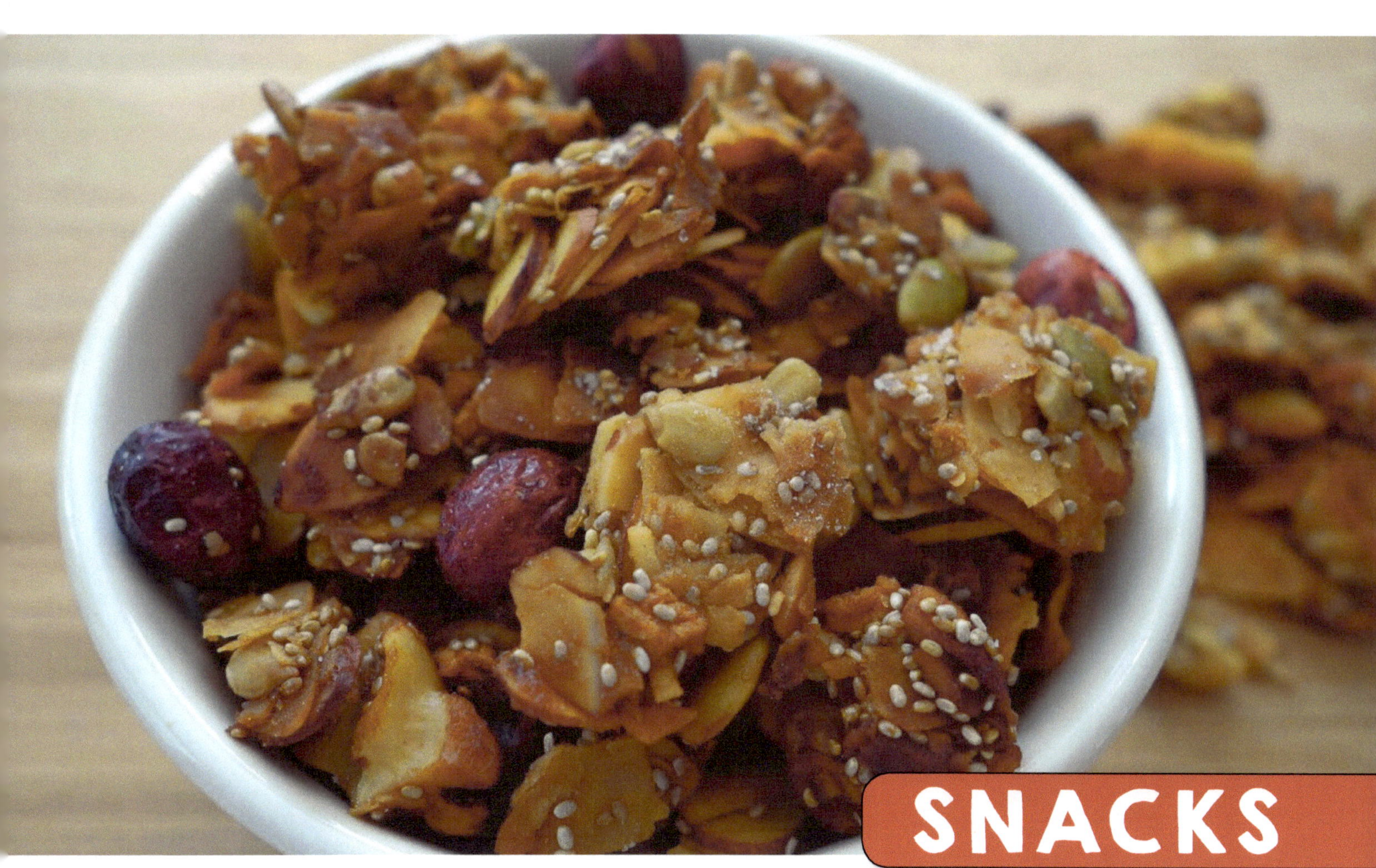

SNACKS

Honey Mustard Kale Chips

INGREDIENTS

- 4 – 6 large kale leaves
- 1 tbsp honey
- 1/2 tbsp olive oil
- 1/2 tsp dry mustard
- 1/4 tsp garlic powder

DIRECTIONS

1. Preheat oven to 200 F degrees.
2. Wash the leaves and break into small 2 chunks.
3. Toss the kale chunks in the honey and olive oil.
4. Sprinkle the mustard and garlic powder on top.
5. Stir until evenly covered.
6. Lay out flat on a baking sheet.
7. Bake for 50 minutes, flipping pieces halfway through.

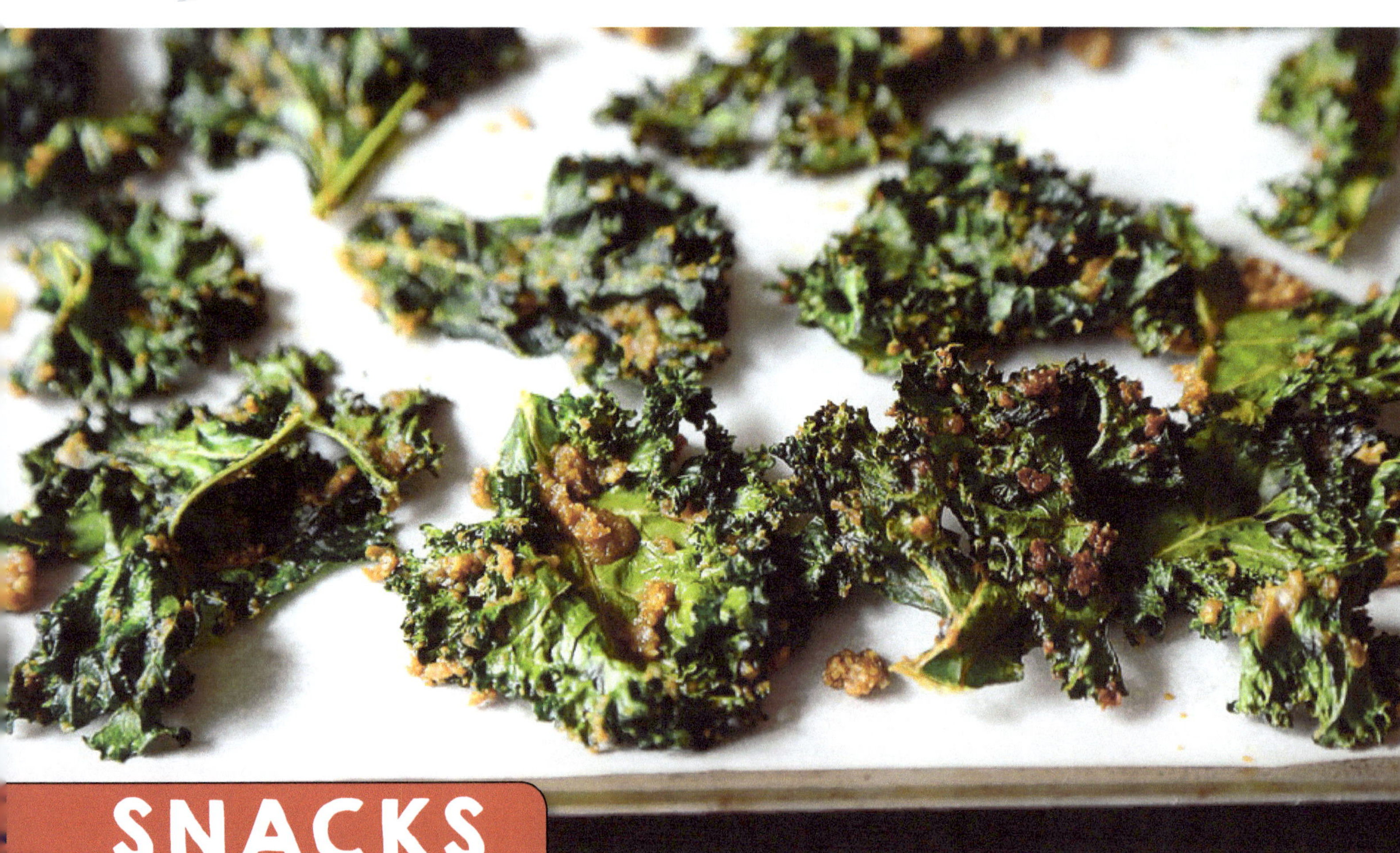

SNACKS

Protein Energy Balls

INGREDIENTS

- 1 1/2 cups rolled oats
- 1/2 cup vanilla protein powder (about 2 scoops)
- 1/2 tsp cinnamon
- 1 Tsp chia seeds
- 1/2 cup smooth natural peanut butter (or any nut butter)
- 3 T raw honey
- 1 tsp vanilla extract
- 1/3 cup unsweetened chocolate chips (optional)
- 2-4 Tbsp liquid (almond milk, cashew milk, water etc...)

DIRECTIONS

1. Add oats, protein powder, and cinnamon and chia seeds to a large bowl.
2. Add in peanut butter, honey and vanilla extract. Stir to combine.
3. Add in chocolate chips if using. Mixture should be slightly sticky but still crumbly.
4. Slowly add in liquid 1 tablespoon at a time and using hands (get dirty!) combine until it comes together in a sticky ball that holds together. If mixture is too dry, add in more liquid but not so much that it won't hold shape.
5. Roll into balls using hands.
6. Place in a container to set in the fridge for at least 30 minutes.
7. Store in fridge until ready to eat.

Make sure it is drippy. If not you may need to add in extra liquid at the end.

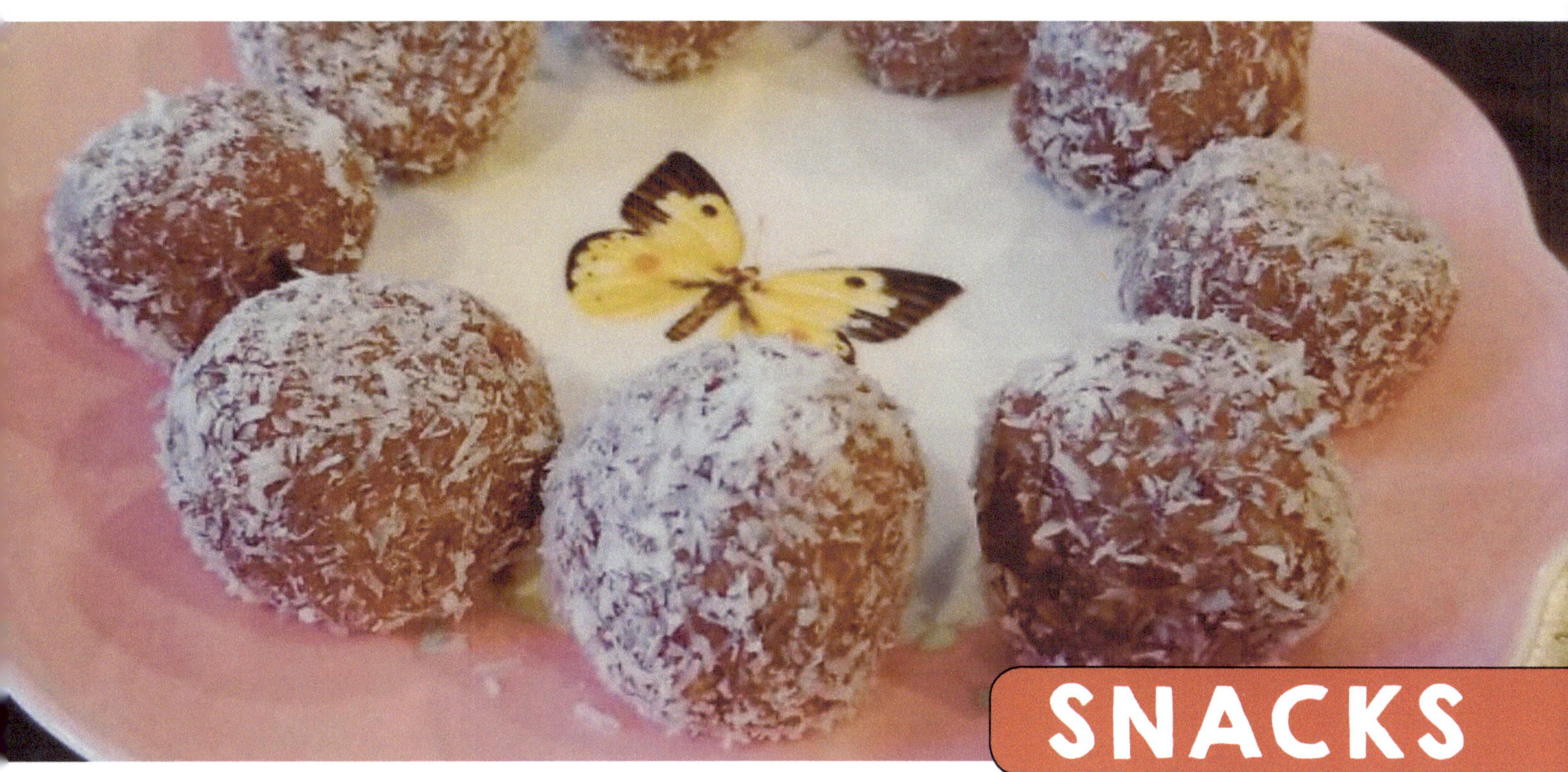

Protein Energy Balls #2

INGREDIENTS

- ¾ cup cashew and almonds
- ¾ cup dates
- 1 scoop vanilla protein powder
- 1 scoop organic coconut flour
- 1 tsp unsweetened coconut flakes

DIRECTIONS

1. Boil dates in water for 10 minutes then drain. Grind nuts first and then add all the ingredients except coconut flakes and blend slowly in blender. Scrape it well.
2. Grease your hand with oil, such as coconut oil. Make half an inch ball. Roll with hand and put it in coconut flakes and roll over.
3. Store in an airtight container.

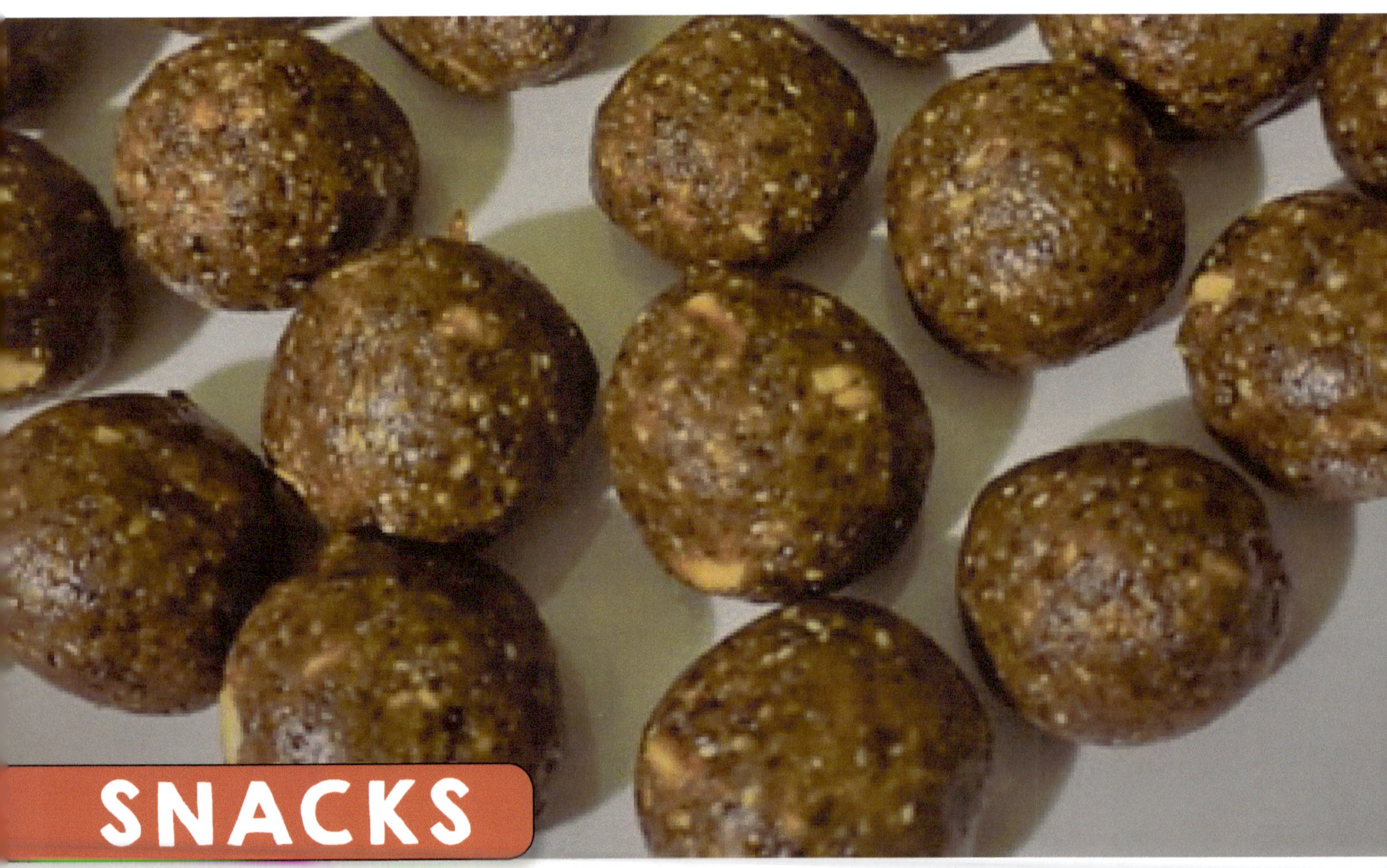

Spicy Roasted Chickpeas (Chana)

INGREDIENTS

- 1 can chickpeas
- ½ tsp Salt
- ½ tsp red chili
- ½ tsp dry mango powder

DIRECTIONS

1. Drain can of chickpeas fully and dry with a clean towel.
2. Heat oven to 400F. Roast the chickpeas for 20 minutes, tossing them around halfway through. Take them out and cool them completely. Then re-bake them at 400F for 10-15 minutes, tossing frequently, until it is crunchy and golden. Cool them completely before storing them.
3. Sprinkle with spices.
4. Drizzle fresh lemon juice just before serving (optional)

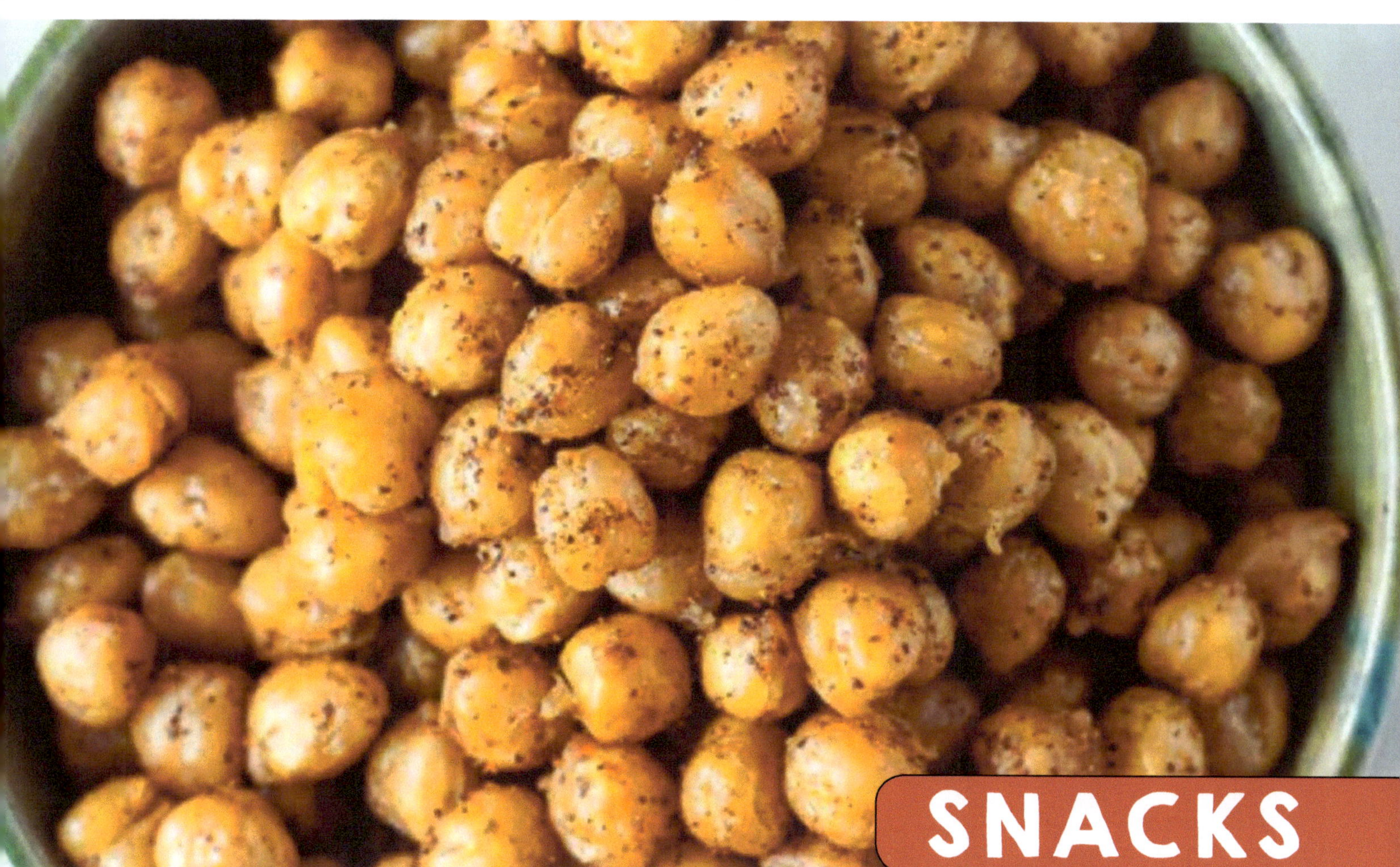

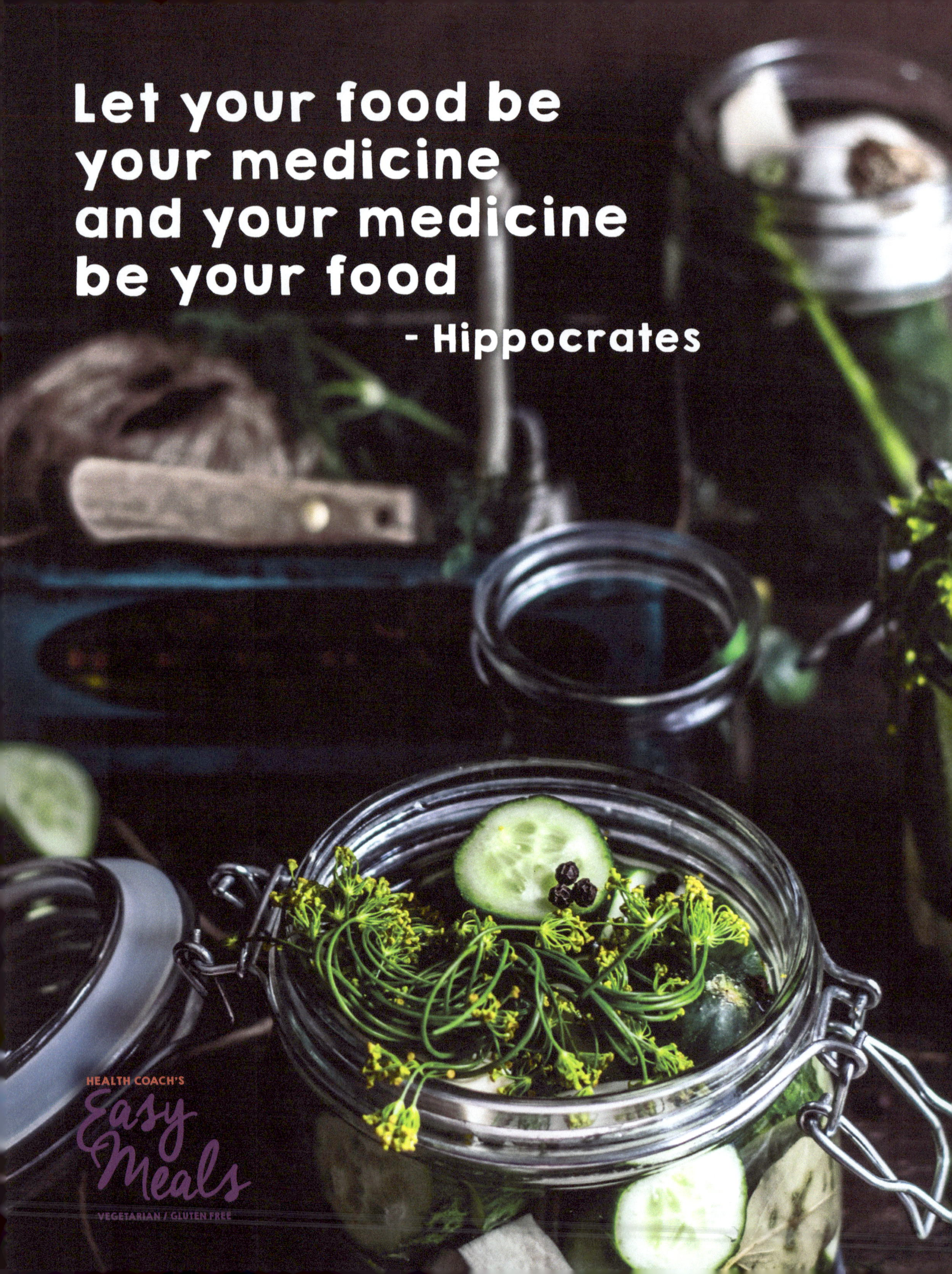

Let your food be
your medicine
and your medicine
be your food

- Hippocrates

HEALTH COACH'S
Easy
Meals
VEGETARIAN / GLUTEN FREE

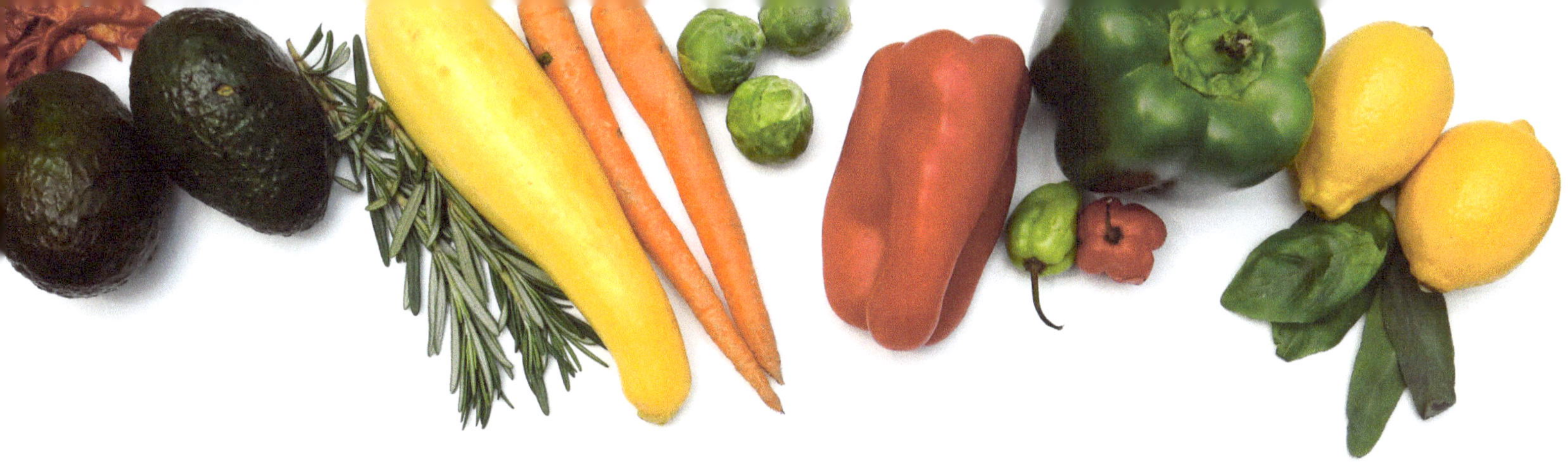

SALADS

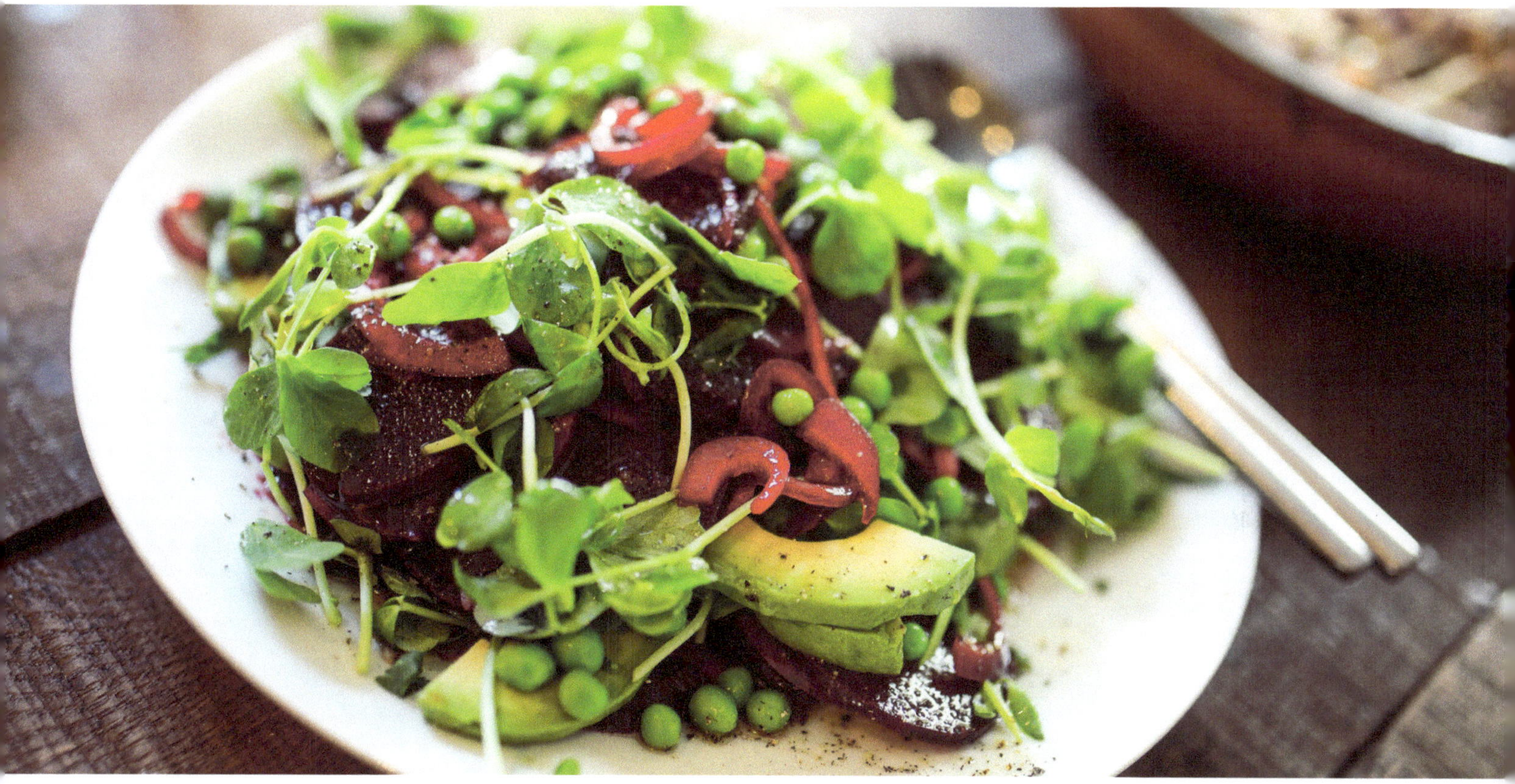

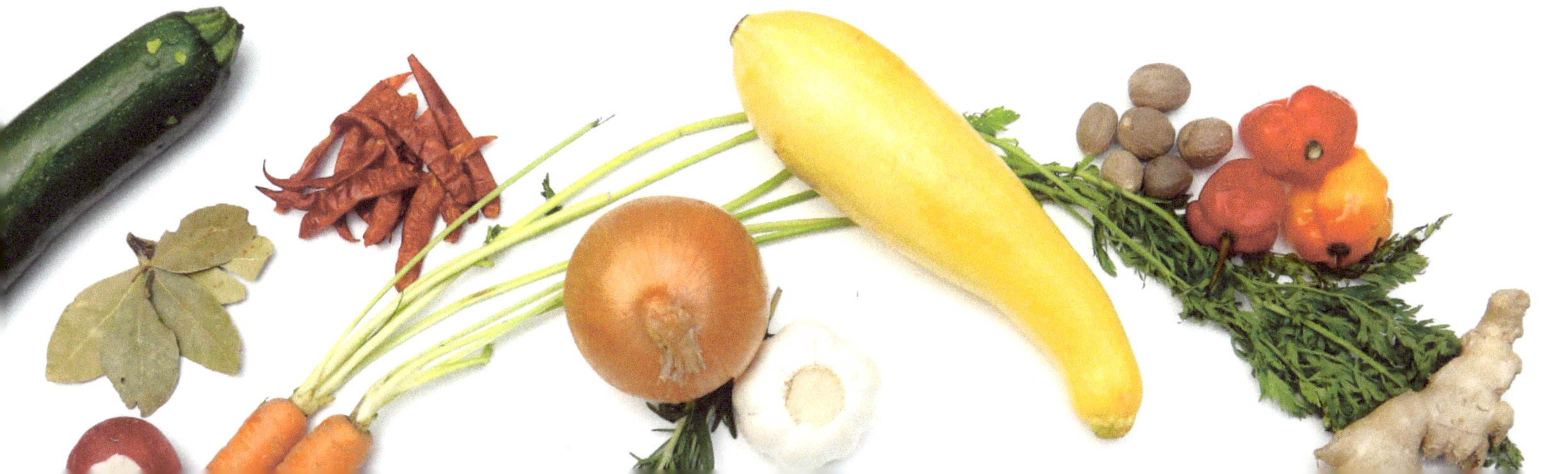

Avocado Bean Salad

INGREDIENTS

- 1 15-ounce can of black beans, drained and rinsed
- 40z of boiled corn kernels
- 1 red bell pepper, seeded and chopped
- 1 orange bell pepper, seeded and chopped
- 1 avocado, cubed
- ¼ cup fresh cilantro, chopped

INGREDIENTS FOR DRESSING

- 1 lime, juiced
- 2 tbsp olive oil
- Pinch salt and pepper

DIRECTIONS

1. Wash and prepare ingredients, and then add all salad ingredients to a large salad bowl
2. In a small dish, mix together dressing ingredients and use a fork or a whisk to combine together thoroughly
3. Pour the salad dressing over the salad and mix together with a fork or spoon.
4. Serve the salad

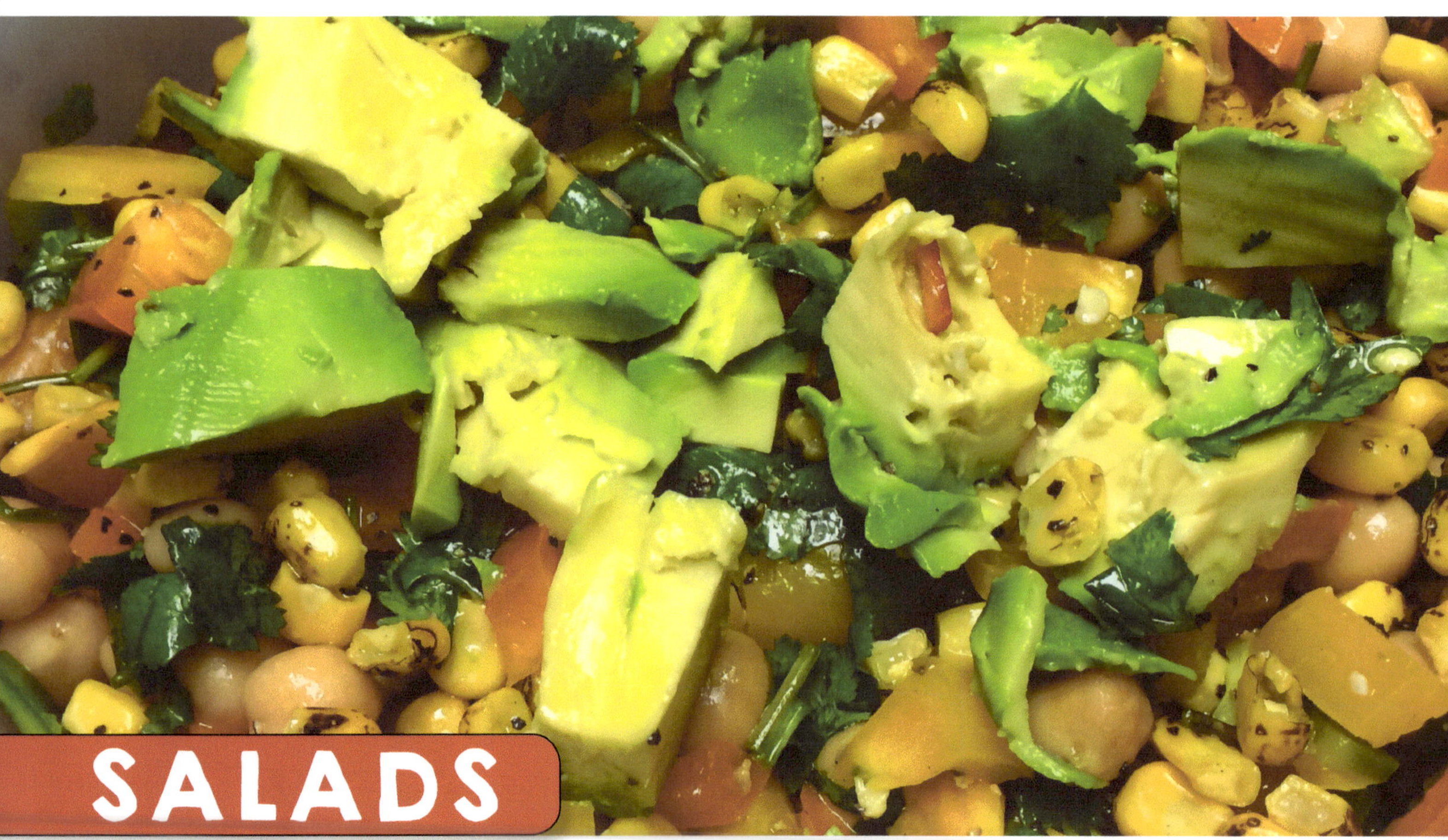

Sprouted Lentils (Moong Dal) Salad

INGREDIENTS

- 1 cup boiled chickpeas
- 1 cup sprouted cooked green gram
- 1 cup chopped onion
- 1 cup chopped tomatoes
- 1/2 cup chopped cilantro
- 2 tsp grated ginger
- 1 tsp each : salt, Asfoedita (Hing) , red chili, mango powder and cumin
- 1 tbs olive oil
- 1 cup chopped cucumber

DIRECTIONS

- Heat oil. Add cumin seeds. Wait until they start to crackle.
  Add onion and ginger and stir for one minute. Add tomatoes and all the spices and stir.
- Add sprouted gram and chickpeas and stir for one minute.
  Cool and add chopped coriander and cucumber.
- Serve cold or hot.

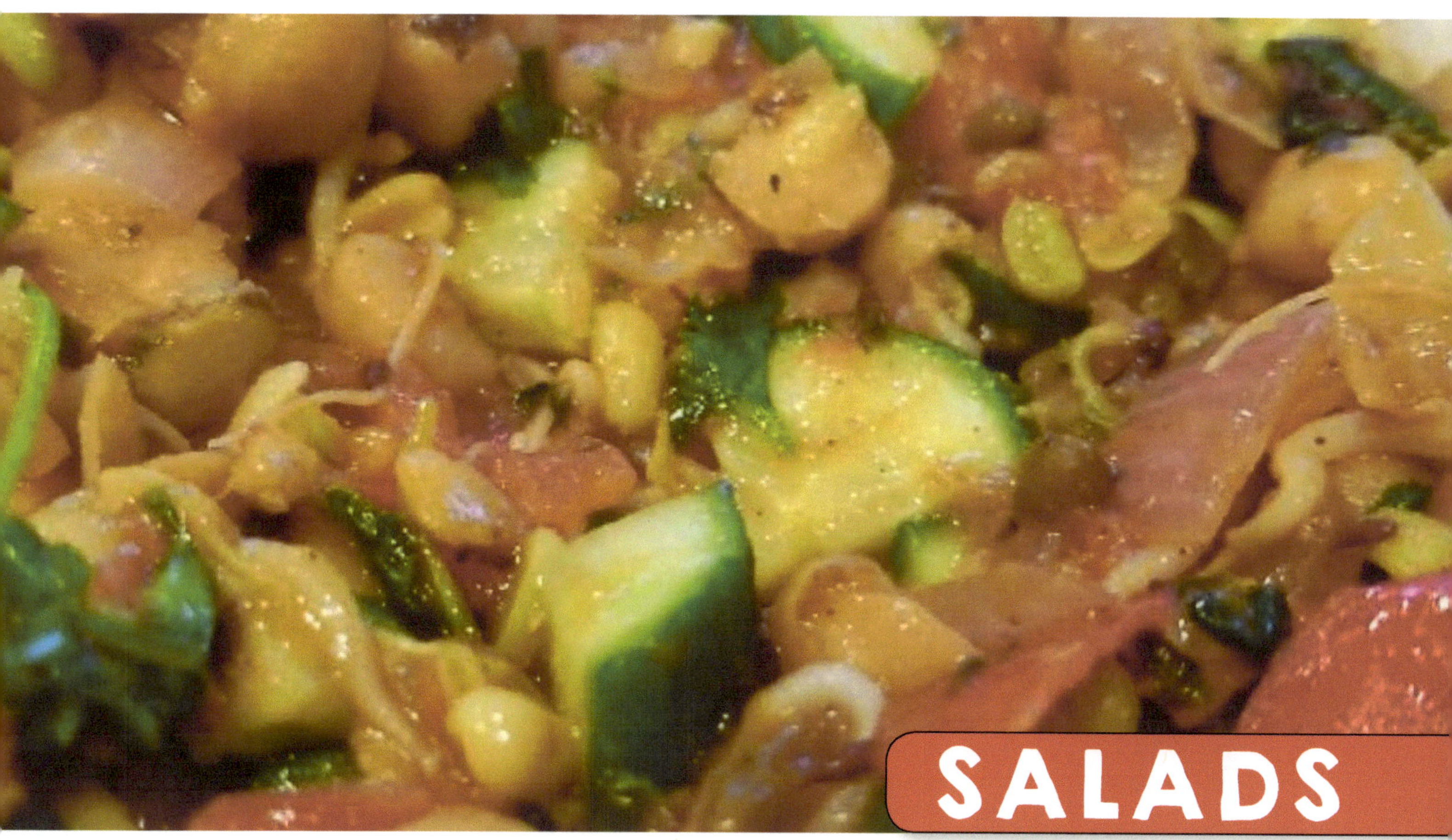

Vegetable Salad

INGREDIENTS

- 3 cups of Fresh Romaine Lettuce
- 1 cup fresh spinach leaves
- ¼ cup red bell pepper sliced
- 3 Mushrooms, sliced

VINAGRETTE DRESSING
INGREDIENTS

¾ cup extra-virgin olive oil
¼ cup white wine or white balmasic vinegar
1 tsp honey
¼ tsp salt
1/8 tsp freshly ground black pepper

DIRECTIONS

Place all the ingrdients in a container with a tight-fitting lid, cover, shake vigorously to combine. The oil and vinegar will emulsify, but then separate over time. Simply shake again before using. The mixture can be stored in a cool, dark place, but if you refrigerate it the oil will thicken a bit and hold the emulsification better after shaking.

DIRECTIONS

- Mix all the ingredients

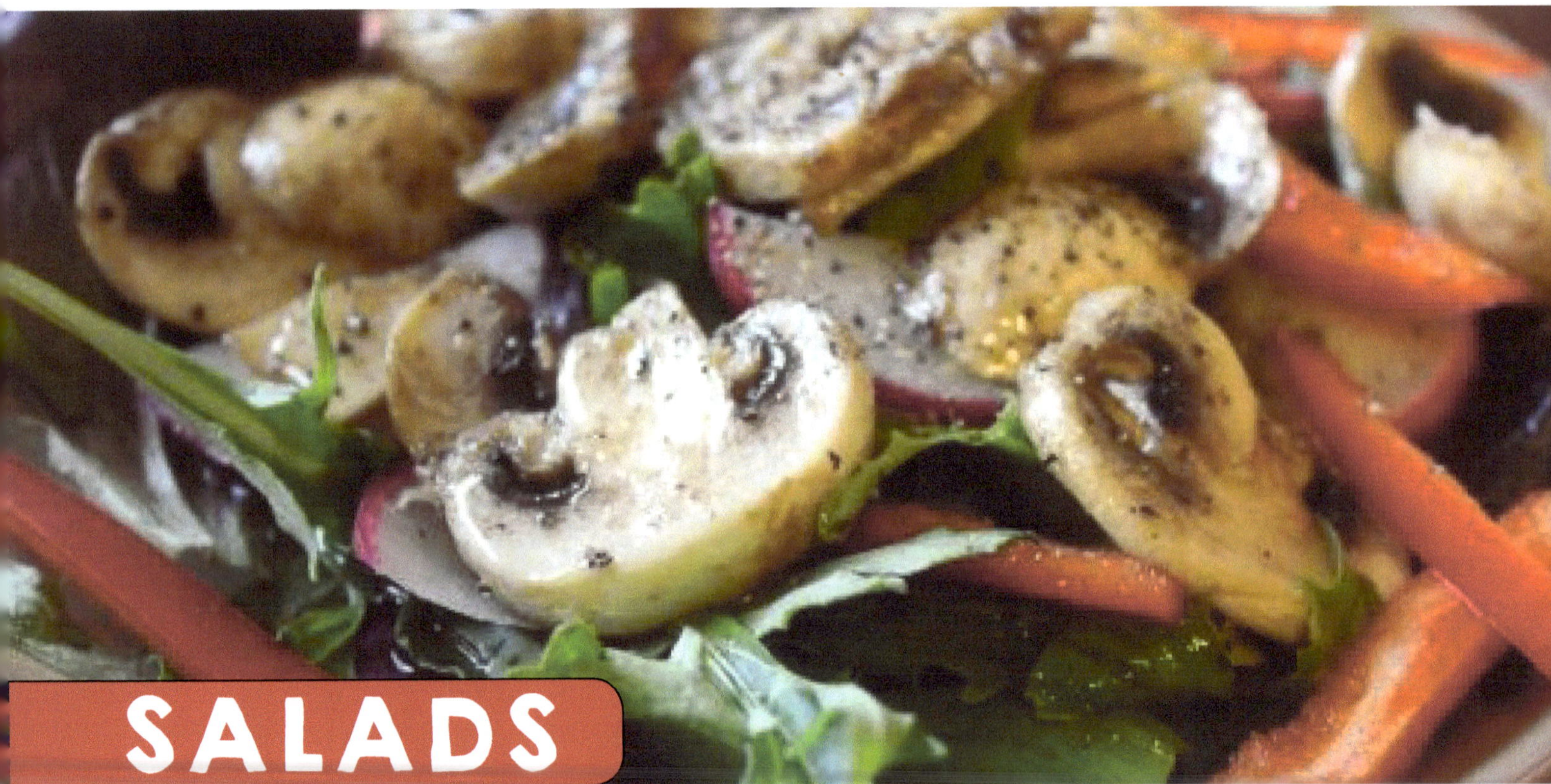

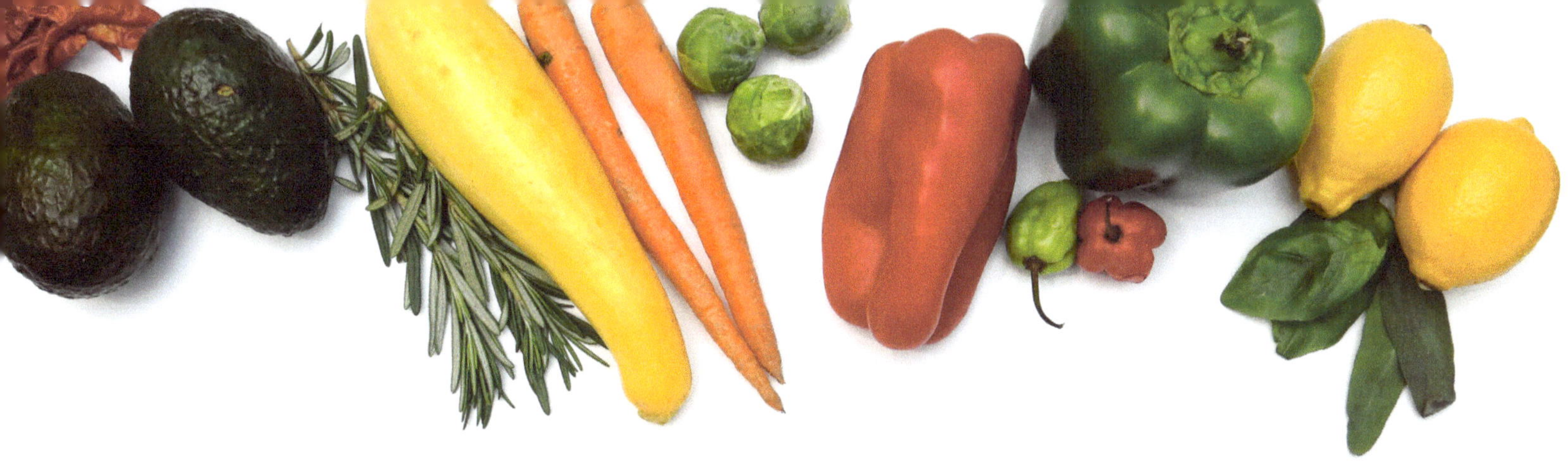

ENTREES

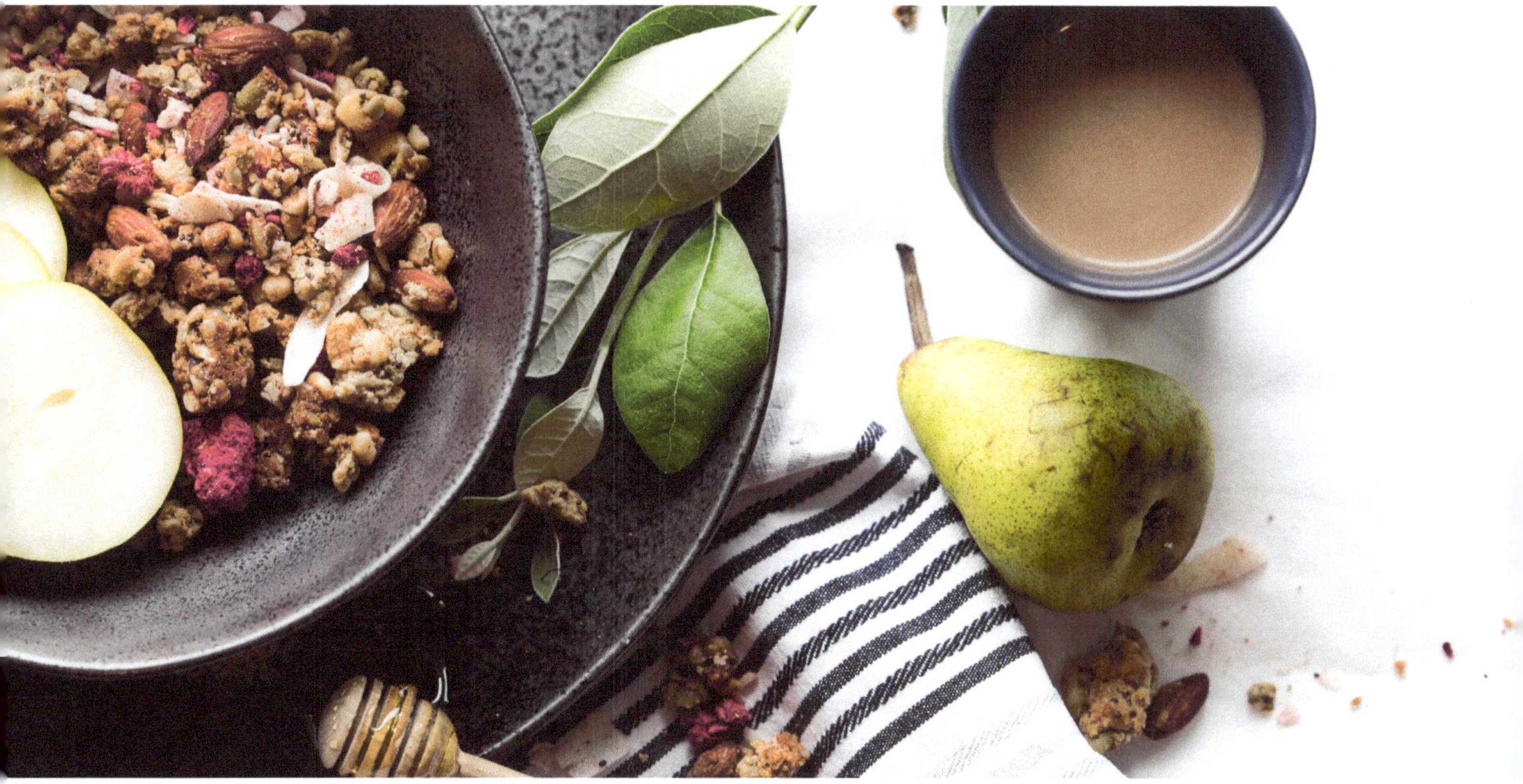

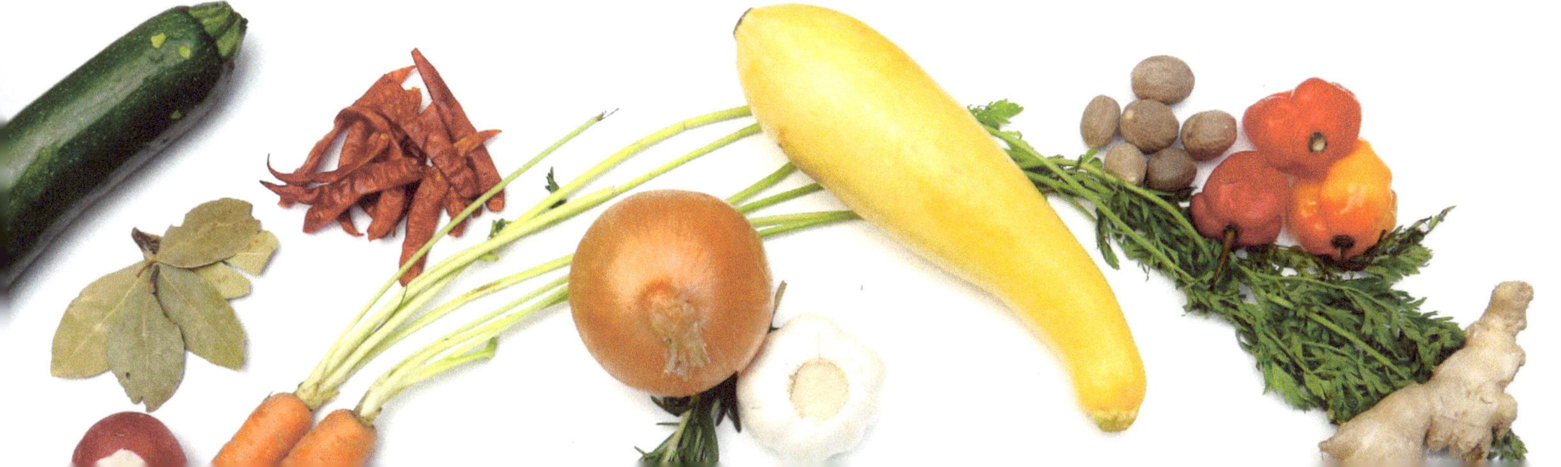

Tofu Scramble

INGREDIENTS

- 1 8oz package of firm tofu
- 1 small red onion
- 2 garlic cloves (minced)
- 1 teaspoon of minced ginger
- 1 tsp cumin seeds
- 1-2 green chili or 1 small jalapeno
- 1 tsp ground turmeric
- 1 tbs coconut oil or ghee (clarified butter)
- Salt n pepper to taste
- Cilantro for garnish

DIRECTIONS

1. Heat oil in a pan and add cumin seeds when oil is warm
2. When cumin seeds start to splutter add chopped onions
3. Slightly brown onions
4. Add green chili, garlic and ginger – cook 2-3 minutes
5. Add turmeric, salt and pepper and cook another 2 minutes
6. Add crumbled tofu and mix well so all tofu is covered in spices
7. Cook on medium heat for 5 minutes stirring often
8. Turn off heat – serve garnished with fresh chopped cilantro

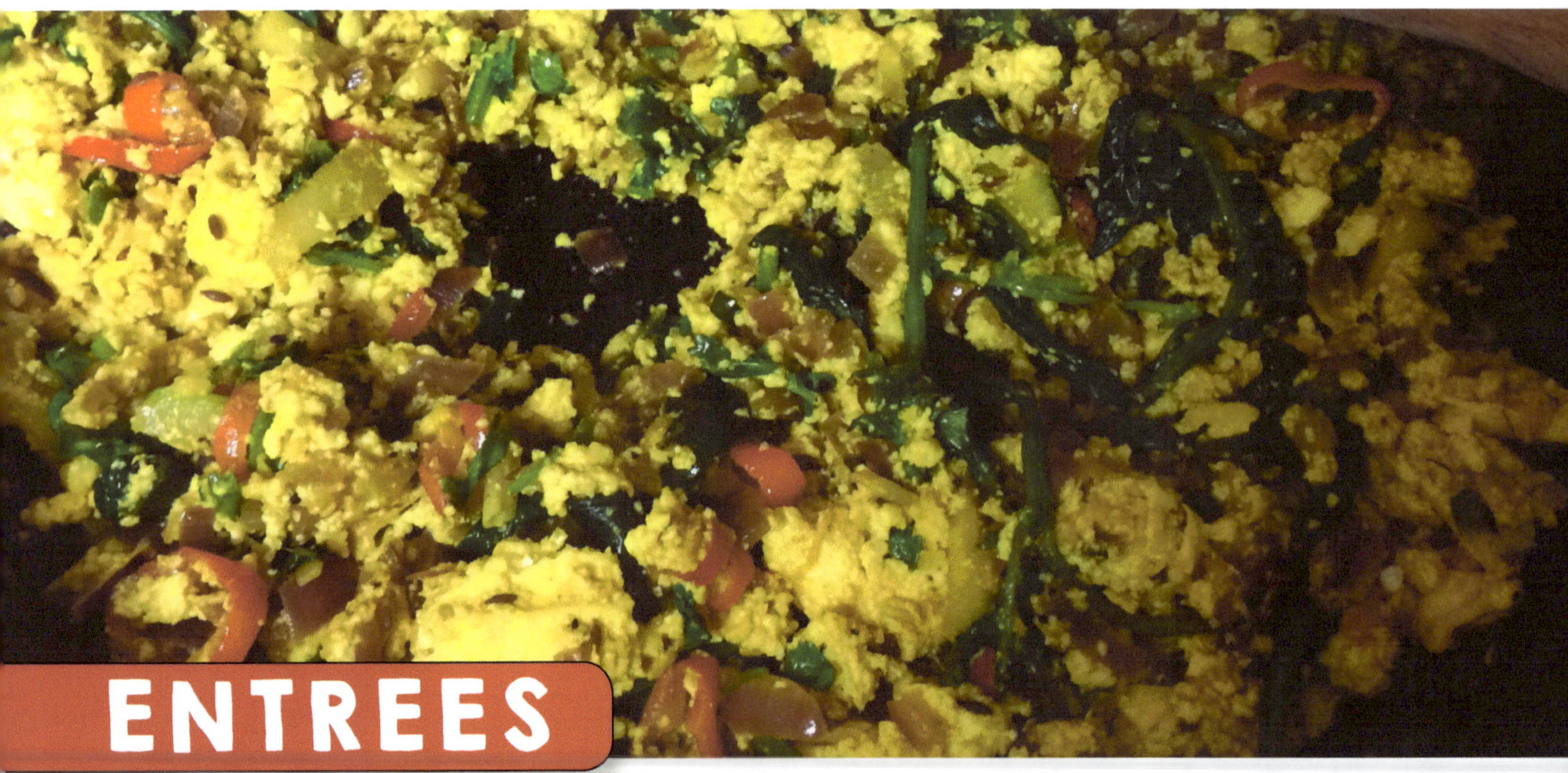

ENTREES

Zucchini Stir Fry

INGREDIENTS

- 1 tablespoon coconut oil
- 1 teaspoon black mustard seeds
- 1 white onion, finely chopped
- 1-2 chili peppers, minced
- 20 fresh curry leaves
- 1 cup grated coconut
- ¼ teaspoon chili powder (or a pinch of cayenne)
- 1 teaspoon turmeric powder
- 1 teaspoon salt
- 4 – 5 cups grated zucchini
- Cilantro for garnish (optional)

DIRECTIONS

1. Melt the coconut oil in a skillet and add the mustard seeds.
2. When the mustard seeds start to splutter, add the onion, chili pepper, curry leaves, grated coconut and spices. Stir for a couple minutes and then add zucchini and stir-fry.
3. Cook on low heat for about ten minutes while stirring occasionally.
4. Serve garnished with Cilantro

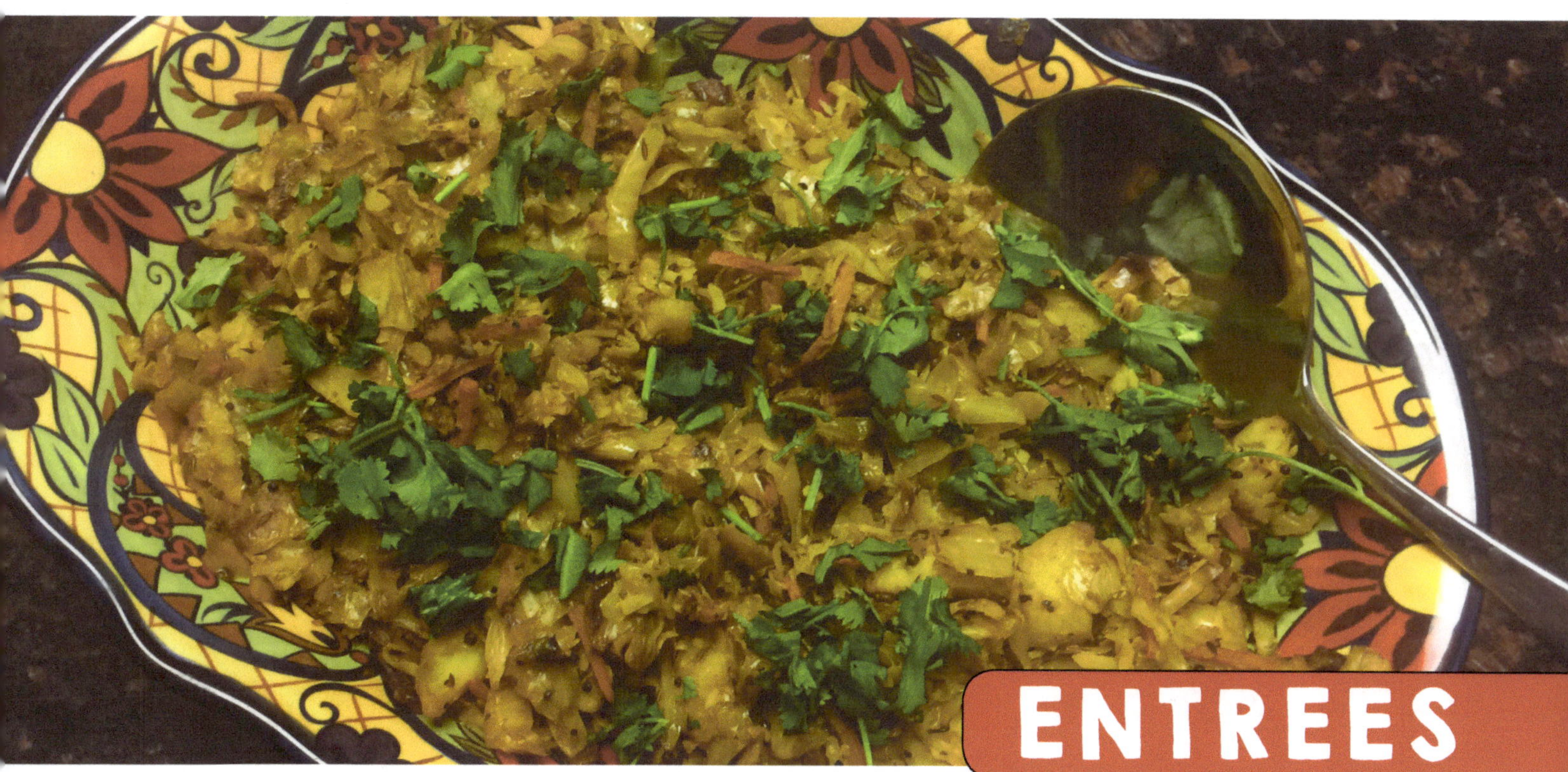

Tofu and Sweet Potato Curry

INGREDIENTS

- 1 brown onion, finely diced
- 2 garlic cloves, minced
- 4 tbsp. red curry paste
- 2 cups soy milk
- 1 cup water
- 1 sweet potato, peeled and cut into small cubes
- 1 carrot, peeled, cut in half lengthwise and finely sliced
- ¼ tsp salt
- ¼ tsp cayenne pepper
- 1 tsp cumin
- ½ tsp turmeric
- 1 14oz can chickpeas, drained and rinsed
- 8oz extra firm tofu, cubed
- cilantro, to garnish

DIRECTIONS

- Heat the olive oil in a large pot, add the garlic and onion and sauté for 5 minutes.
- Add the red curry paste and stir till coated. Add the soy milk, water, sweet potato, carrot and spices and bring to a simmer. Simmer for 15 minutes.
- Add the chickpeas and tofu and simmer for another 5 minutes.
- Serve the curry with brown rice and garnish with cilantro. Serve immediately.

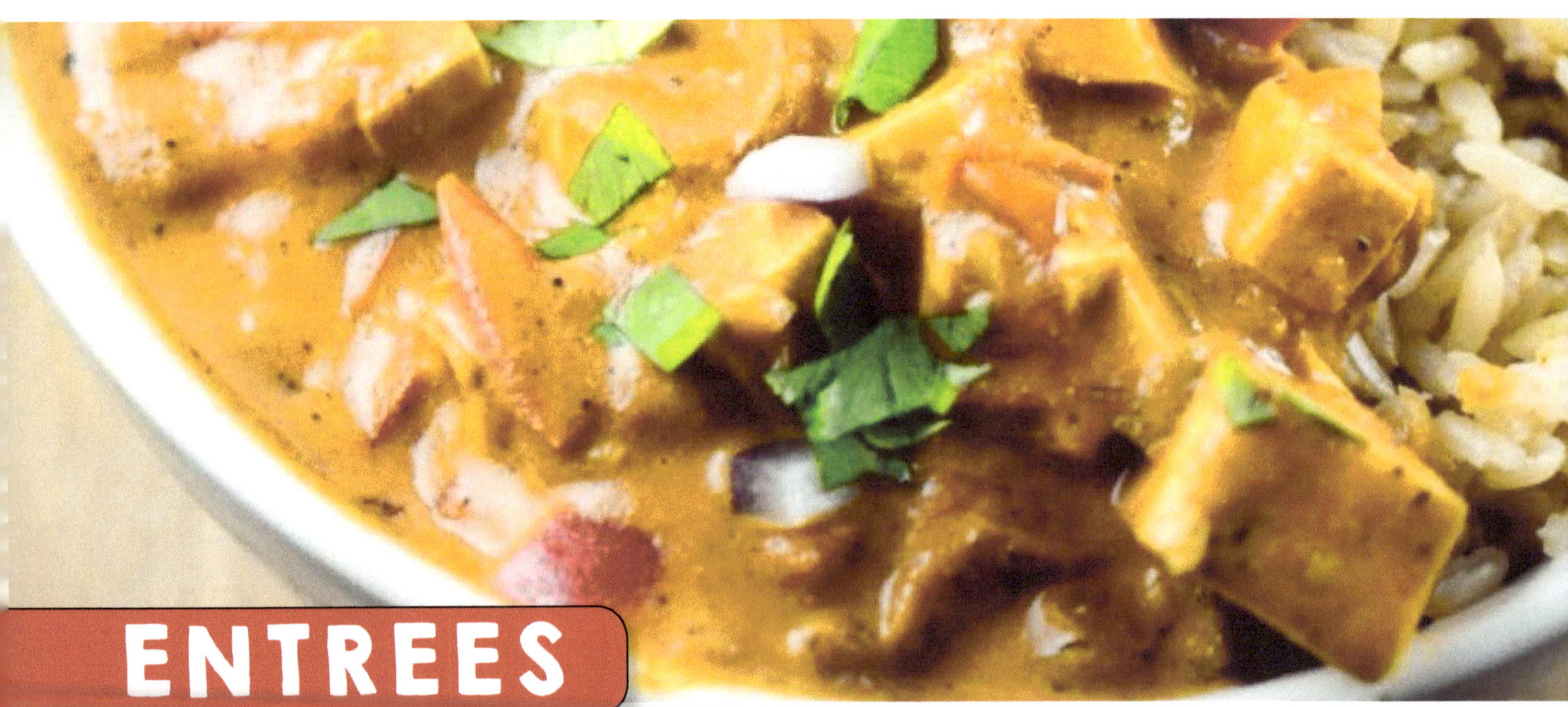

Vegetarian Chili

INGREDIENTS

- 2 tbs olive oil
- 1 1/2 cups chopped red onions
- 1 cup chopped green bell peppers
- 3 cloves of minced garlic
- 2 Thai green chili and minced,
- depending upon taste
- 1/2 medium zucchini, stem ends trimmed and cut into small dice
- 1 cup chopped celery (about 3 stalks)
- 1/2 tablespoons chili powder
- 1/2 tablespoon ground coriander
- 1/2 teaspoon of cumin powder
- 1 teaspoon dried oregano
- 1 teaspoon dried thyme
- 1 inch fresh ginger
- 1/4 teaspoon turmeric
- 1 1/4 teaspoons salt
- 1 teaspoon garam masala (all spice)
- 4 large tomatoes chopped
- 1/3 cup of cooked black beans or canned beans rinsed and drained
- 1/3 cup of cooked chickpea or canned beans, rinsed and drained
- 1/3 cup of cooked Kidney beans or canned beans, rinsed and drained
- 1 1/2 cup vegetable stock, or water
- 2 tablespoon chopped fresh cilantro leaves
- Diced avocado for garnish

DIRECTIONS

- In a large, heavy pot, heat the oil over medium-high heat. Add the onions, fry for 3 minutes then add green chili peppers, bell peppers and celery and fry for another 3 minutes.
- Then add ginger-garlic paste stir for about 2 minutes and add the remaining ingredients
- Reduce the heat to medium-low and simmer, stirring occasionally, for about 30 minutes.
- Remove from heat, sprinkle cilantro to serve hot.

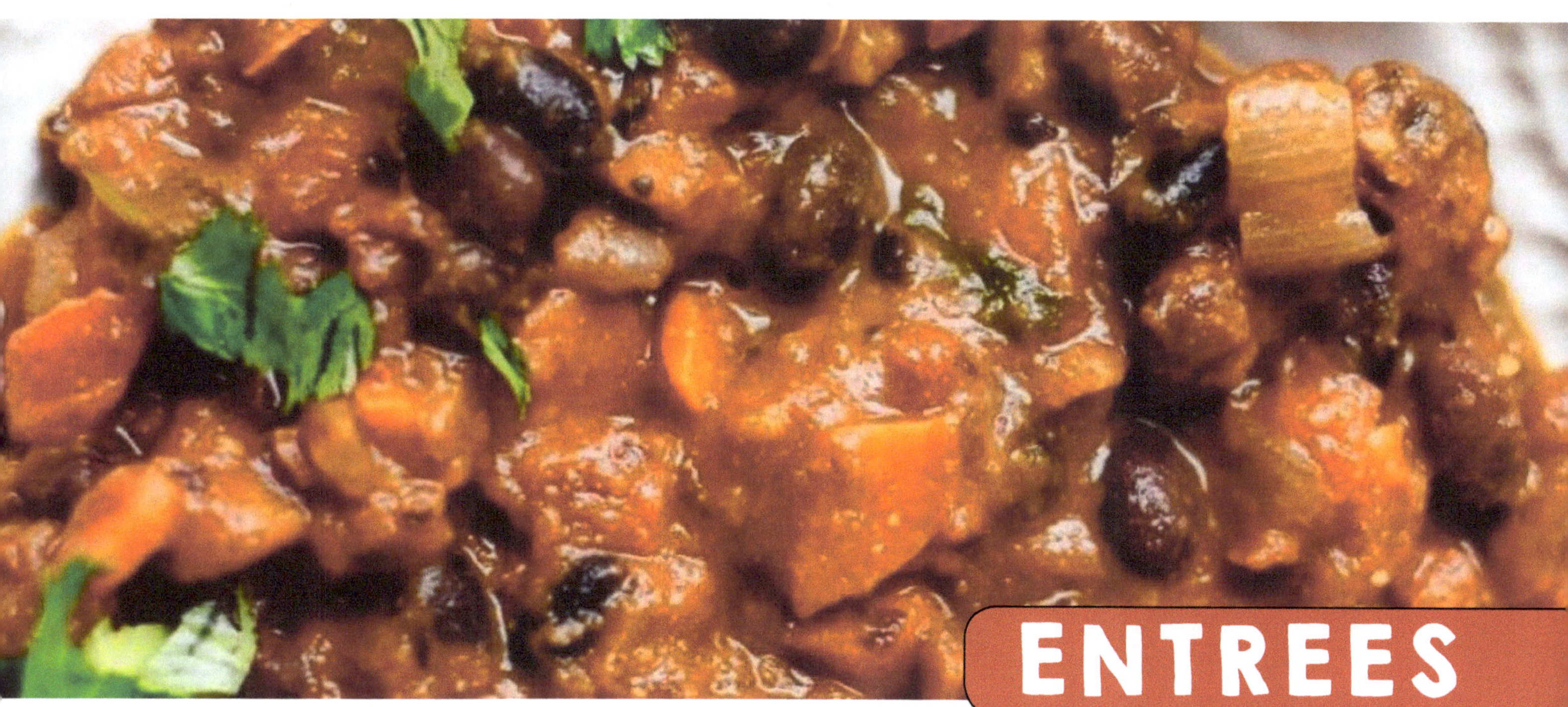

Tofu Grilled / Pan Seared

INGREDIENTS FOR MARINADE

- 1 tablespoon Asian sesame oil
- ¼ cup soy sauce
- 2 tablespoons mirin (sweet Japanese rice wine)
- 1 tablespoon rice wine vinegar
- 1 tablespoon minced or grated fresh ginger

INGREDIENTS FOR TOFU

- 1 pound firm tofu
- 1 tablespoon olive oil
- Additional soy sauce or marinade for topping

DIRECTIONS

- Combine all of the marinade ingredients in a 2-quart bowl. Whisk together well.
- Drain the tofu and pat dry with paper towels. Slice into 1/2-inch thick slabs, and blot each slab with paper towels. Add to the bowl with the marinade, and gently toss to coat. Cover and refrigerate for 15 minutes to an hour, or for up to a day.
- To pan-fry the tofu, heat the oil over medium-high heat in a large, heavy nonstick skillet. When the oil is hot, add the tofu in one layer (you may have to do this in batches). Cook on one side for one to two minutes, until lightly colored. Using tongs, turn the tofu over and cook for another one to two minutes, or until lightly colored on the other side.
- Remove from the pan, and serve with additional marinade or soy sauce. To grill the tofu, prepare a medium-hot grill. Brush the grill with oil, and grill until grill marks appear, 1 1/2 to 2 minutes per side. Remove from the heat, and serve with additional marinade or soy sauce.

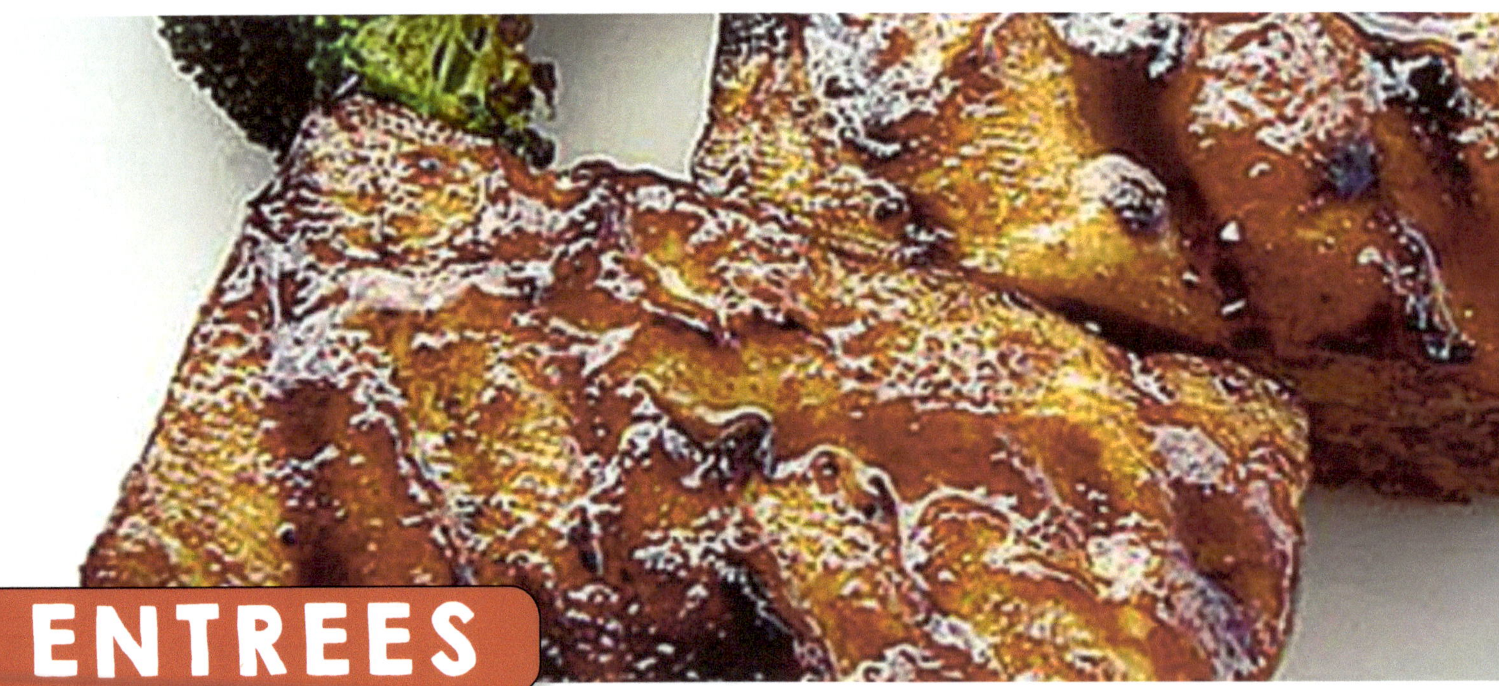

ENTREES

Chana Pindi (Chick Peas)

INGREDIENTS

- Chickpeas (chana) soaked overnight
- 1 tbs dried pomegranate seeds
- 2 Tea bags
- Salt to taste
- 1/2 tsp Turmeric powder
- 1 1/2 Red chili powder
- 1/2 Dry mango powder (amchur)
- 4 tbs clarified butter (ghee) or coconut oil
- 1 1/2 Cumin seeds
- 2 medium onions chopped
- 2tbs Ginger and garlic paste
- 2 tbs Cumin powder
- 2 tbs Coriander powder
- 2 medium tomatoes quartered and 4-6 green chilies slit
- 1 tsp Garam masala powder (all spice)

DIRECTIONS

- Take soaked chick peas in a deep pan. Add tea bags and salt and cook till soft.
- Once cooked remove the tea bags.
- Dry roast pomegranate seeds, half the turmeric powder, half the red chili powder, mango powder. This is the chana masala.
- Heat three tablespoons ghee in an iron skillet and add one teaspoon cumin seeds .
- Add onions and sauté till golden brown.
- Add ginger paste, garlic paste, red chili powder, remaining turmeric powder, cumin powder, coriander powder and pomegranate seeds and continue to sauté
- Add boiled chickpeas, salt and some water and mix.
- Meanwhile heat one-tablespoon ghee in a pan, add the remaining cumin seeds and tomatoes. Add slit green chilies and a little salt and toss.
- Stir and press the tomatoes lightly. Add a little water and cook for two minutes.
- Add to the chana along with Chana masala and garam masala.
- Stir to mix well and cook for fifteen to twenty minutes on low heat. Serve hot.

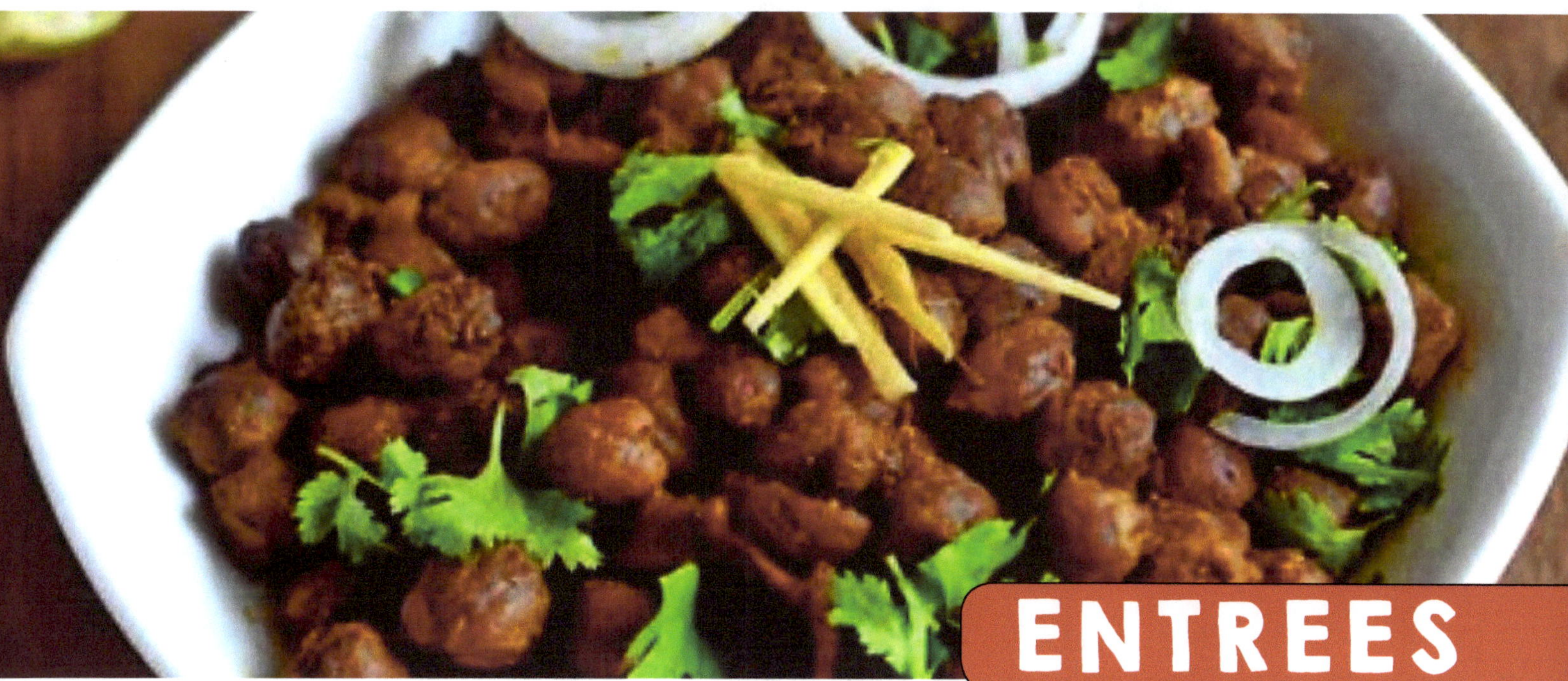

Mixed Greens Curry

INGREDIENTS

- 3 Tbsp Ghee or coconut oil
- 1 ½ Tsp cumin seeds
- 1 chile pepper diced
- 1 cup water
- 1 lb spinach, rinsed and chopped
- 1 lb collard greens, mustard greens or kale, rinsed and roughly chopped
- 1 tsp minced garlic
- 1 tsp grated fresh ginger
- ¼ tsp garam masala
- Salt to taste

DIRECTIONS

- In a deep skilled or dutch oven, heat the ghee over medium high heat. Add cumin seeds and chili pepper and sauté until the seeds start to sputter about 30 seconds. Add the water and enough spinach and greens to fill the skillet, then stir to coat with the ghee. As the spinach and greens start to wilt add the remained until all has been added. Stir in the garlic, ginger, garam, masala and salt.
- Cover and reduce heat to low. Simmer about 20 minutes until dark green and tender stirring occasionally. Remove cover and increase heat to medium and simmer until most liquid has evaporated about 10 minutes. Serve with Roti or Brown Rice or Quinoa Pulao

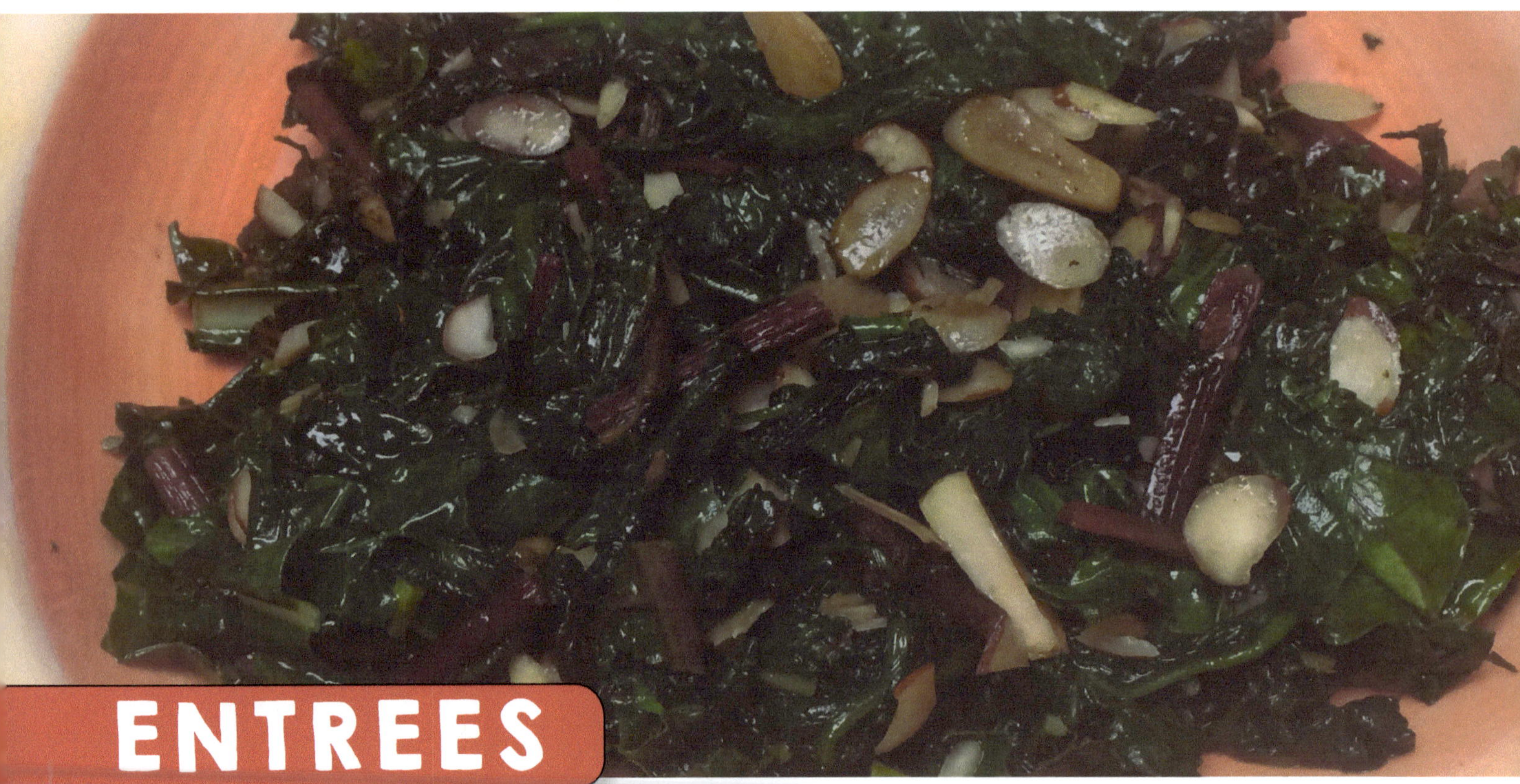

Quinoa Fried Rice

INGREDIENTS

- 2.5 cups cooked quinoa
- 2 teaspoons oil, I used avocado oil
- 1 small red onion, chopped
- 2 garlic cloves, crushed
- 2 green chili, crushed
- ½ inch ginger, crushed
- 1 medium tomato, chopped
- ½ cup cauliflower florets, small
- ¼ cup green peas
- salt, to taste
- juice of 1 lemon
- cilantro/mint, to garnish

WHOLE SPICES

- 1 bay leaf
- 2 black cardamoms
- 2 green cardamoms
- 2 cloves
- 4 black peppercorns
- 1 cinnamon stick

DIRECTIONS

- Heat oil in pan on medium heat. Once the oil is hot, add bay leaf, green cardamom, black cardamom, peppercorns, cinnamon stick and cloves. Saute for 30 seconds till fragrant.
- Add chopped onion and saute for 2 minutes.
- Then add the crushed ginger-garlic-green chili and cook for a minute or so till the raw smell goes away.
- Add chopped tomato and cook for 2 minutes or so.
- Then add all the veggies – cauliflower and peas Also add salt.
- Once the veggies are cooked, add the cooked quinoa.
- Mix everything till well combined. Check salt at this point and adjust to taste.
- Squeeze in some fresh lemon juice and garnish with cilantro or mint

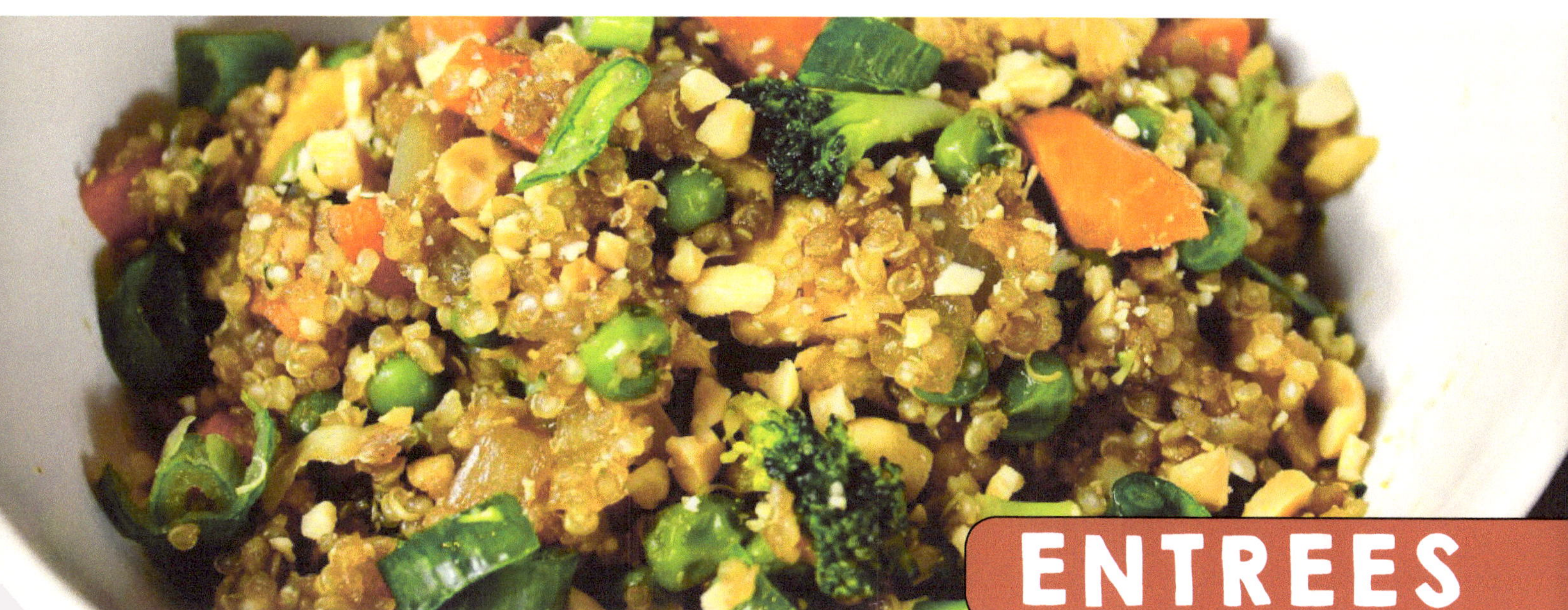

Roti, Naan, Bread

INGREDIENTS

- ½ cup almond flour
- ½ cup tapioca flour
- 1 cup coconut milk
- Salt to taste
- Coconut oil or Ghee (clarified butter)

DIRECTIONS

- Mix all ingredients in a bowl
- Warm some oil in a skillet
- Pour ¼ batter in pan and spread evenly
- Cook for one minute on both sides
- Serve with any vegetable or curry

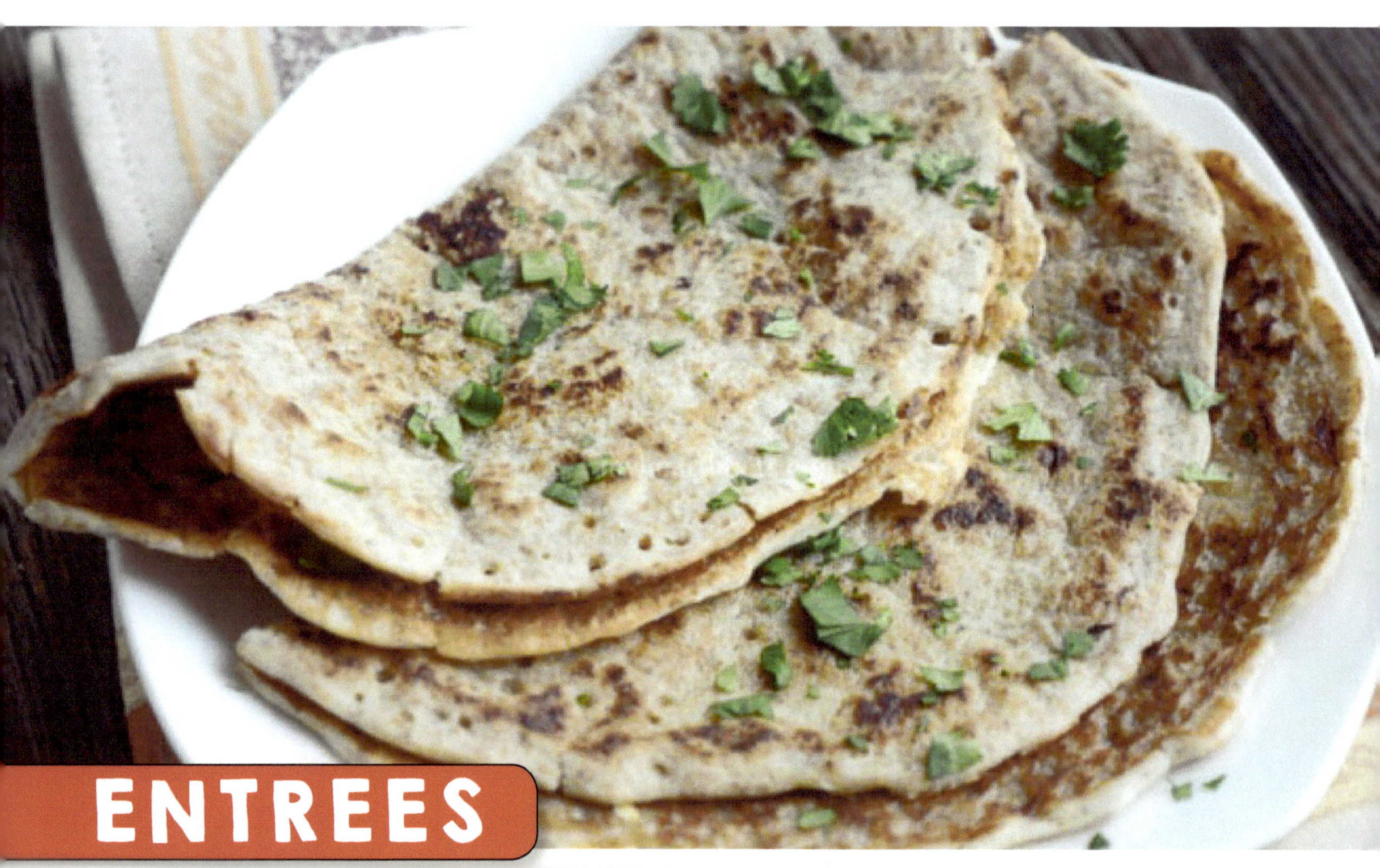

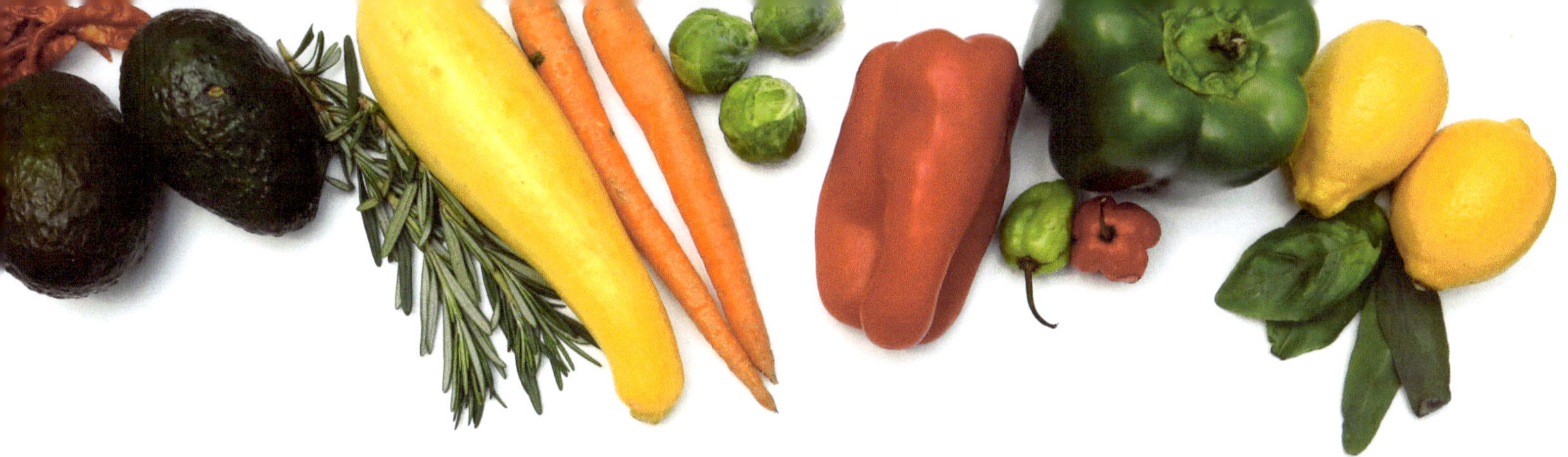

BEVERAGES

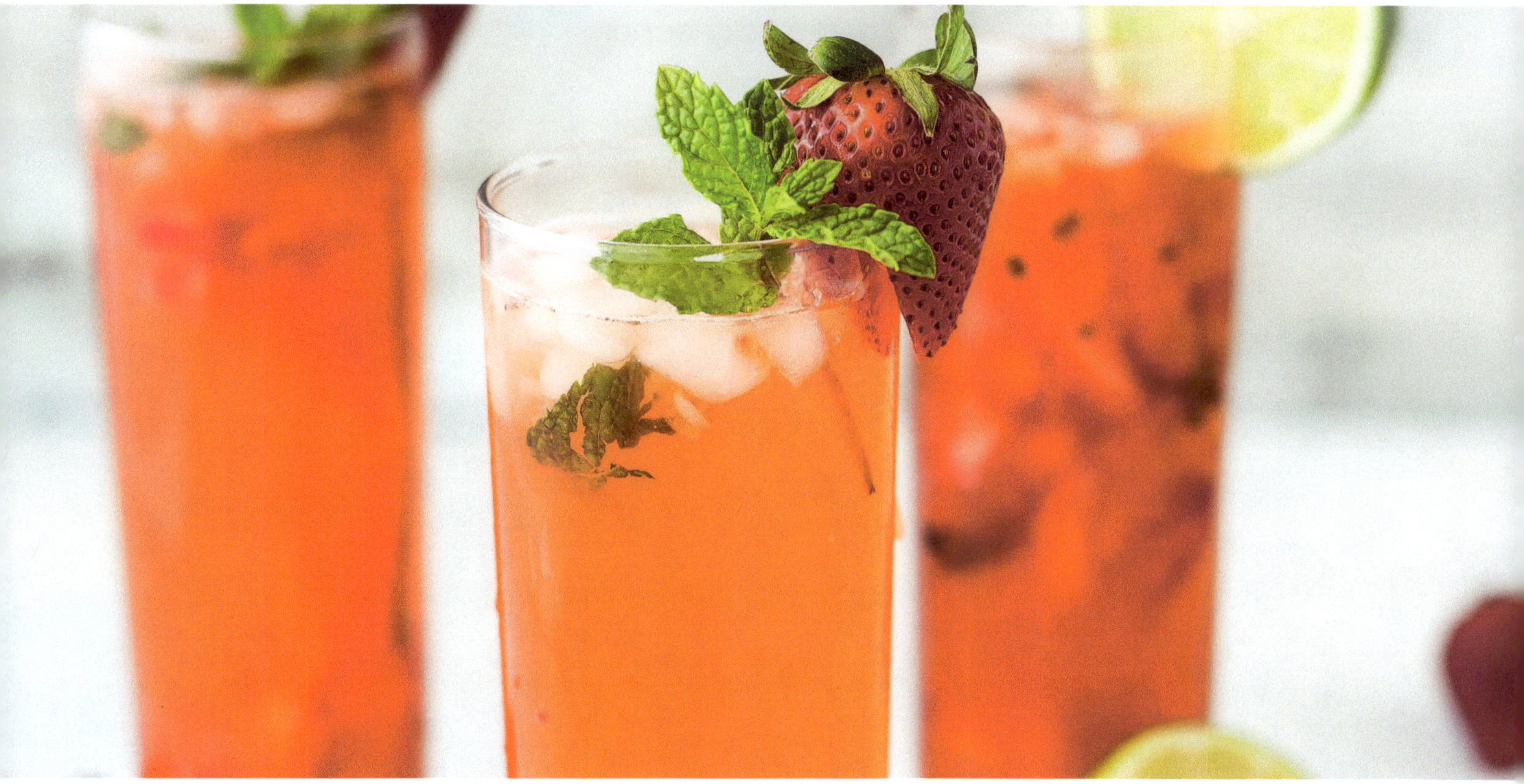

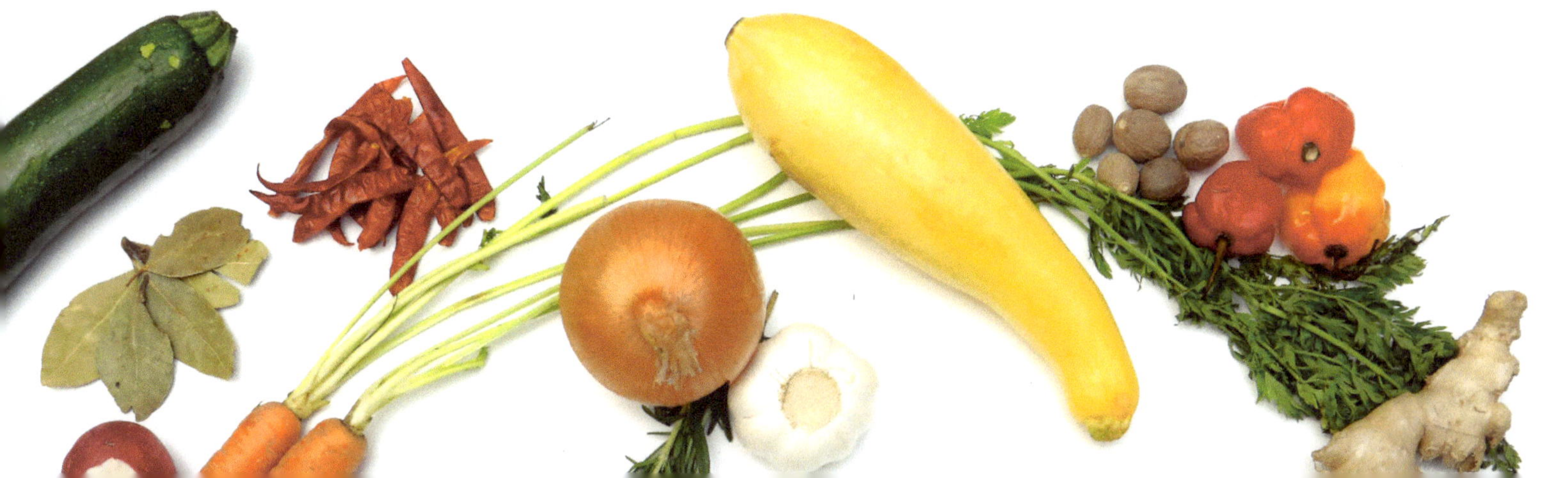

Ginger Turmeric Tea

INGREDIENTS

- 1 tbs grated ginger
- 1 tbs grated turmeric root (or two tablespoons powder turmeric)
- ¼ tsp ground black pepper
- ½ tsp raw honey

DIRECTIONS

- In a small saucepan, bring a cup of water to boil. Turn off the heat and add grated ginger and turmeric.
- Steep with the lid on for 5 minutes.
- Strain the tea and add the honey and black pepper
- Serve hot

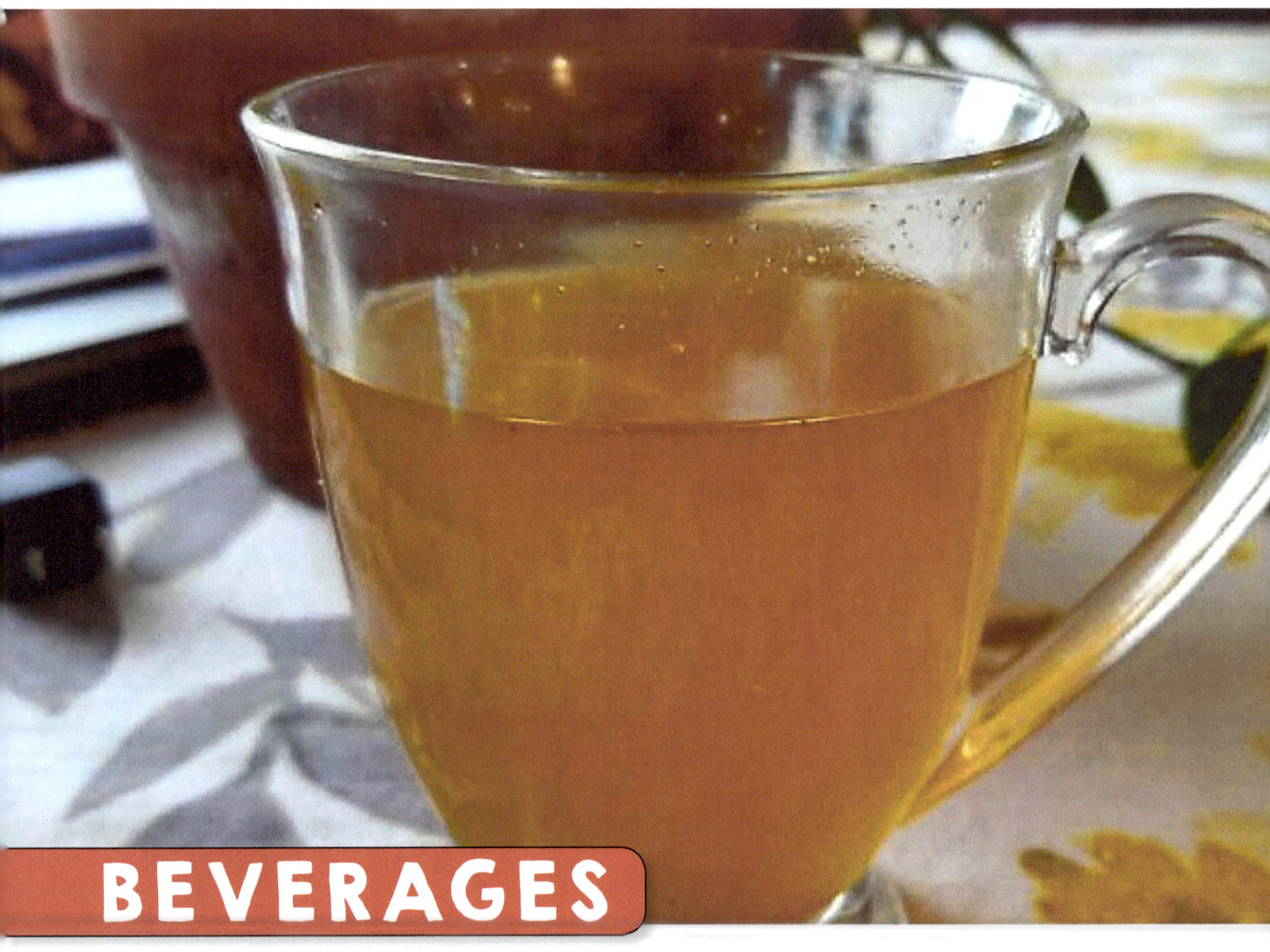

Cashews Smoothie

INGREDIENTS

- 1 cup Cashews
- 1 cup Almond Milk
- 1 Frozen Banana
- 5 Cardamom Pods - just use seeds or use a big pinch of ground cardamom

DIRECTIONS

1. Add all of the ingredients to your blender; secure lid and blend until smooth.
2. Pour into a glass and enjoy!

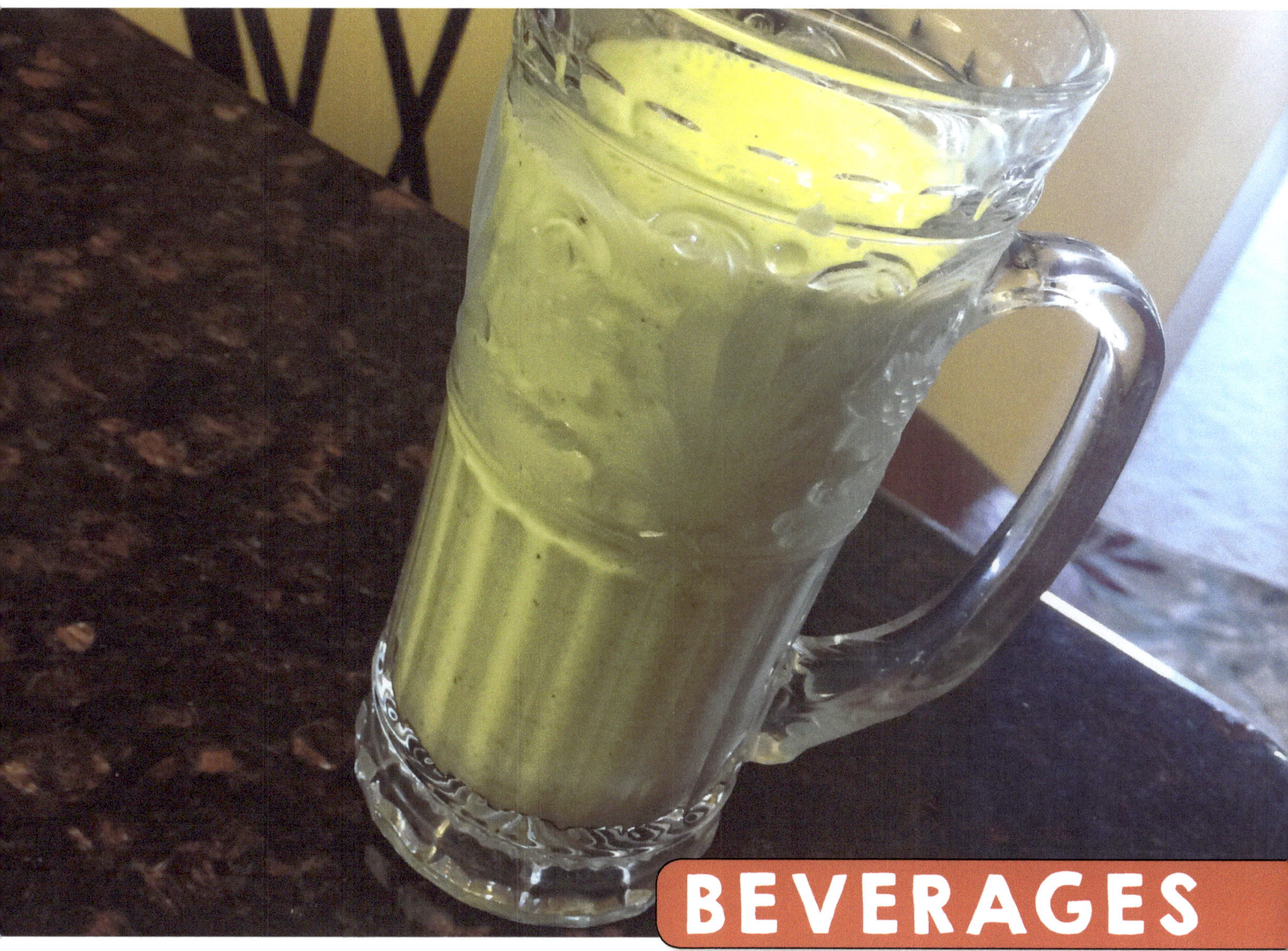

Quick Hot Chocolate

INGREDIENTS

- 1 cup almond milk
- 5-6 dates , soaked overnight and pit removed
- 1 tablespoon Organic Raw Cacao

DIRECTIONS

1. Add all of the ingredients to a blender and blend until smooth.
2. Warm up the chocolate mixture (either on the stovetop or in a microwave) and serve.

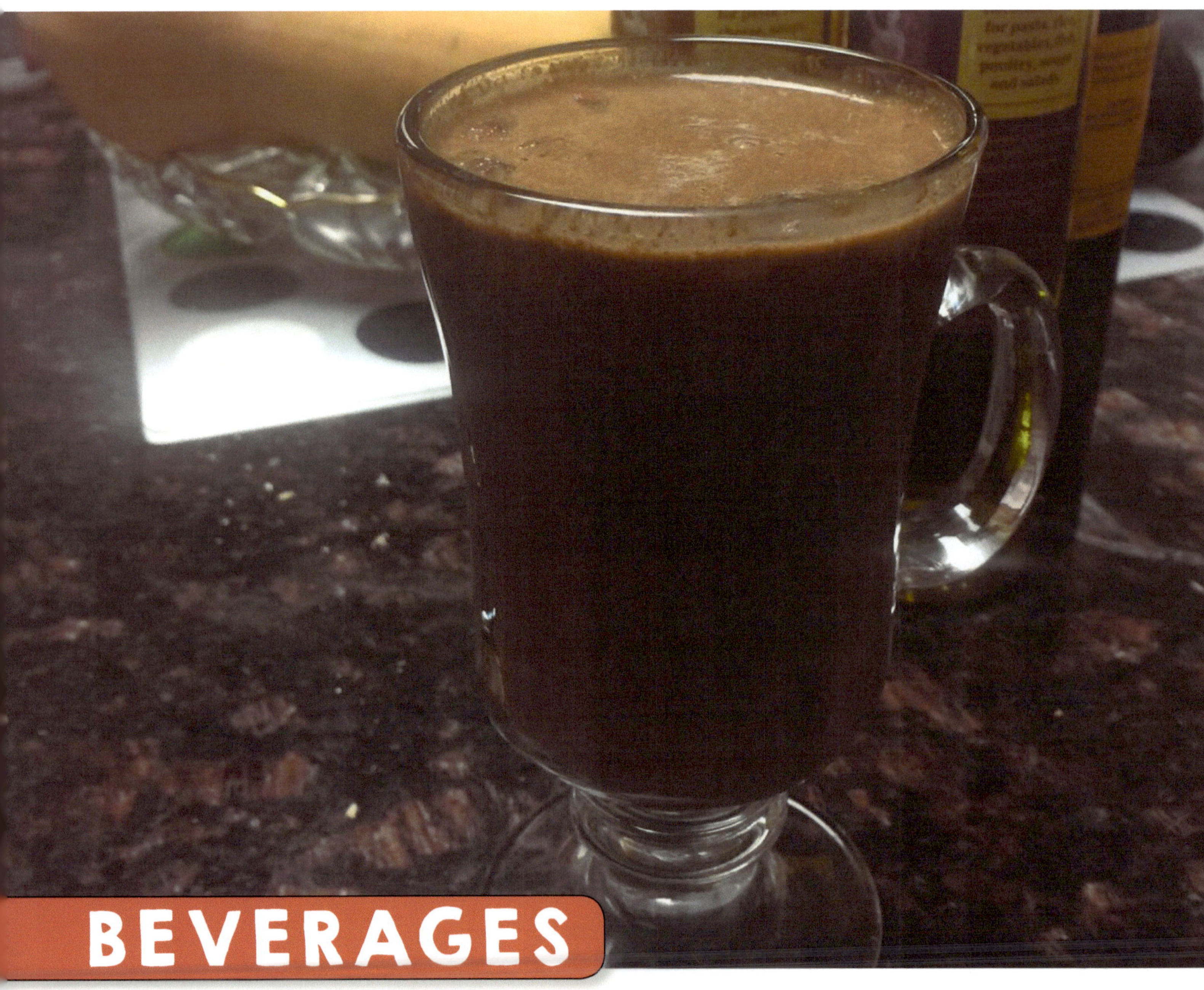

BEVERAGES

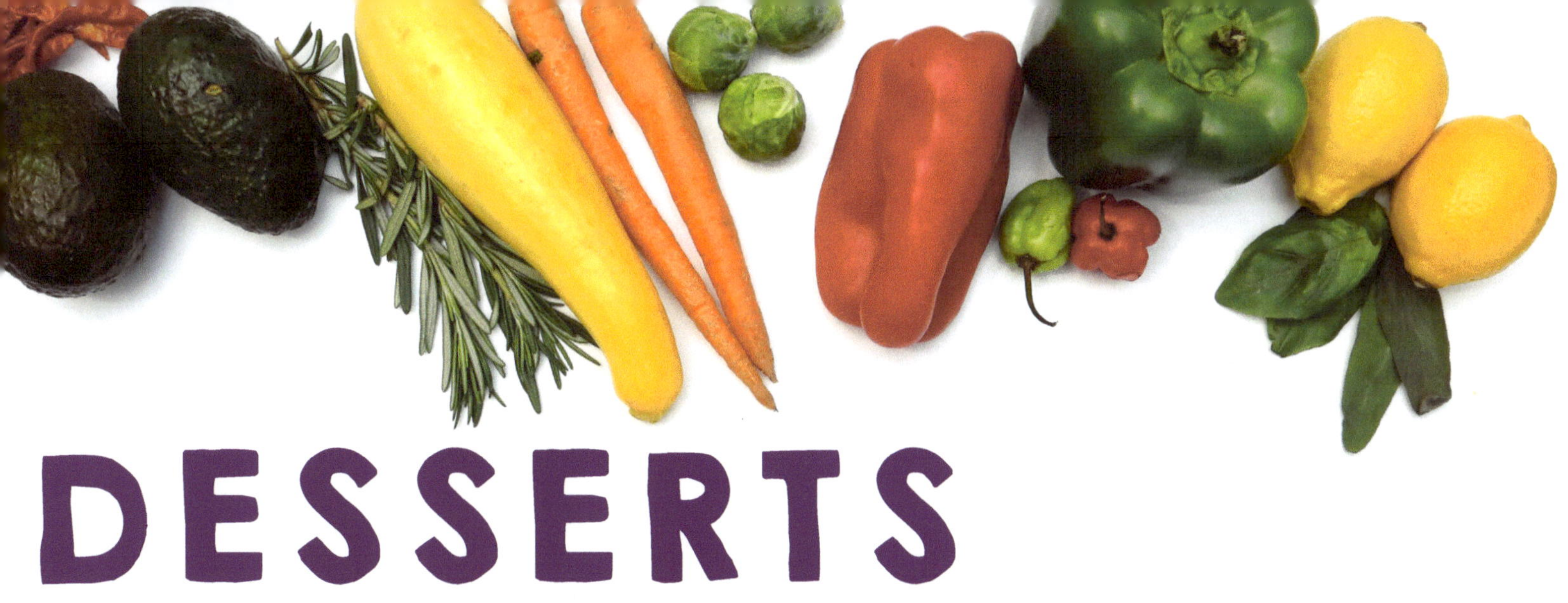

DESSERTS

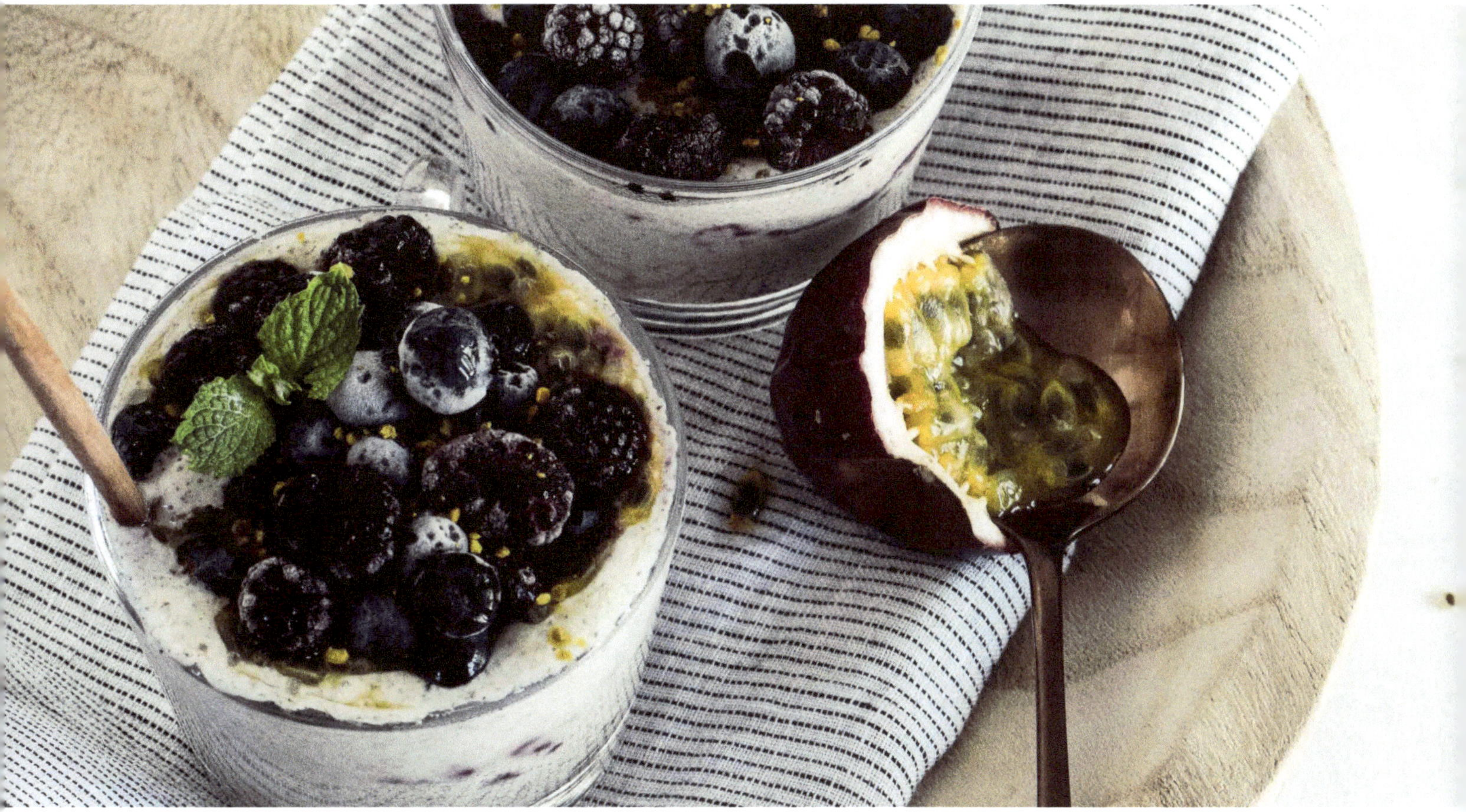

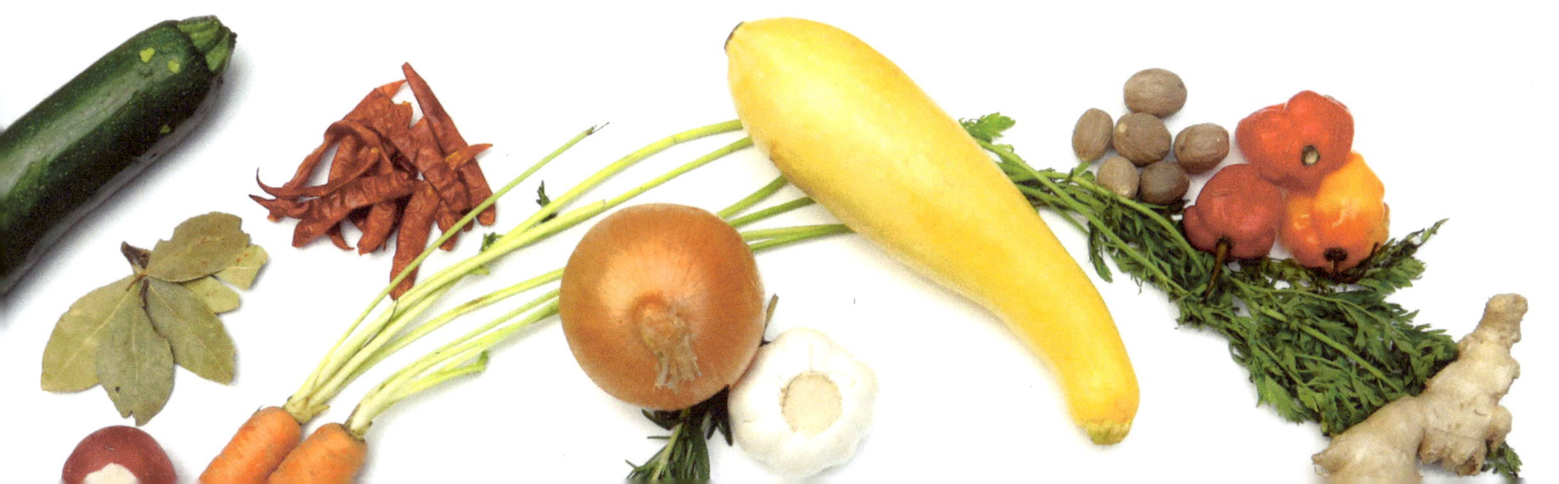

Mango Sorbet

INGREDIENTS

- 4 mangos, diced
- ½ cup honey
- ½ cup water

DIRECTIONS

- Cut mangoes into ½-inch cubes and put on baking sheet. Cover and freeze for a minimum of 4 hours.
- In a food processor, add the frozen mango, water, and honey. Mix until the mixture is smooth.
- Remove from food processor and scoop into tray.
- Freeze for one additional hour.
- Enjoy!

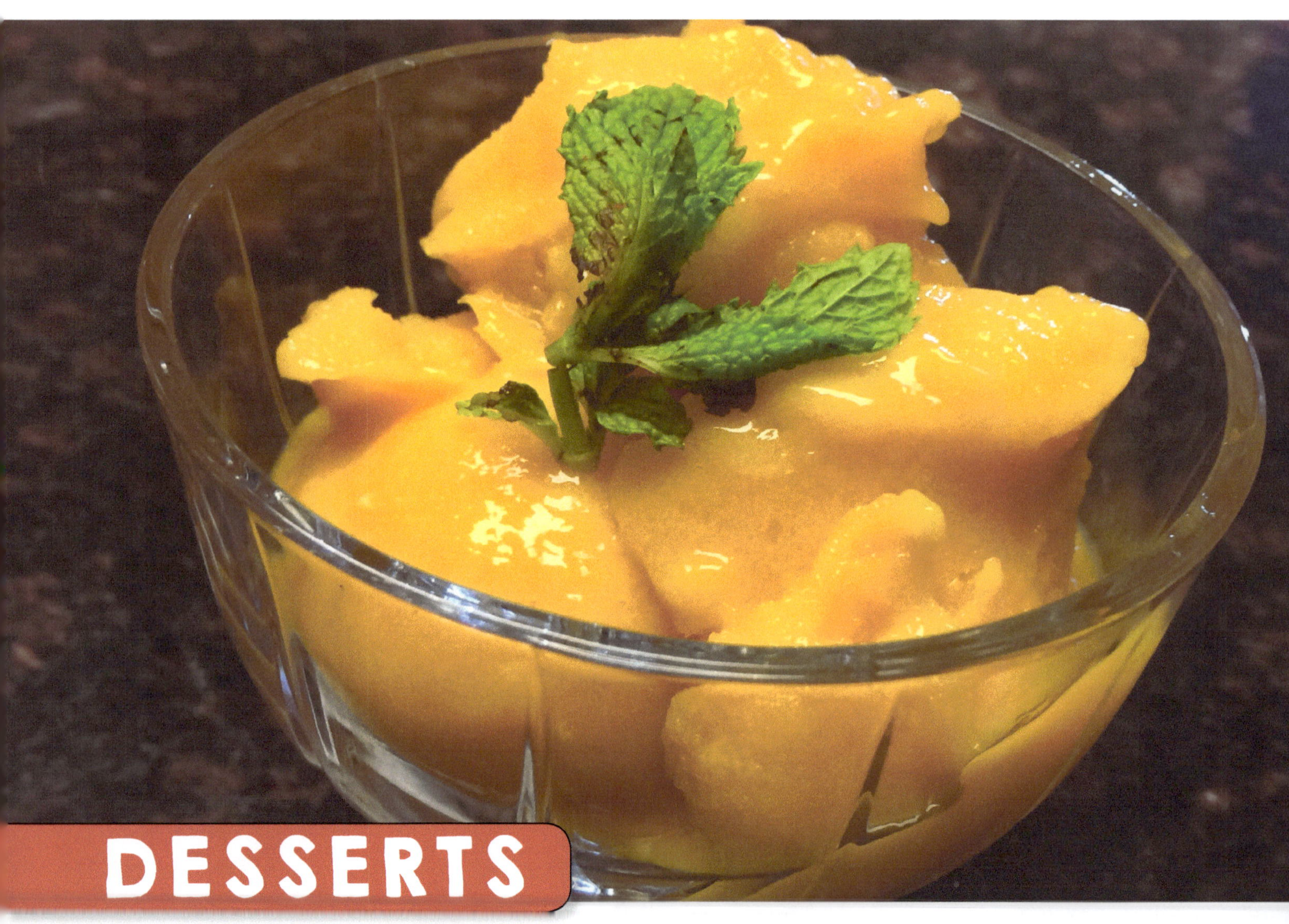

Chia Pudding

INGREDIENTS

- ½ cup Chia seeds
- 2 cups full fat coconut milk
- 1 tsp Vanilla essence
- 1 cup mixed chopped nuts
- 2 tbs Maple Syrup
- 1 scoop Vanilla protein powder

DIRECTIONS

- Mix all the ingredients except chia seeds and blend for 30 seconds.
- Whisk chia in the mixture and pour in a dish and keep in fridge for 4 to 5 hours.
- Serve

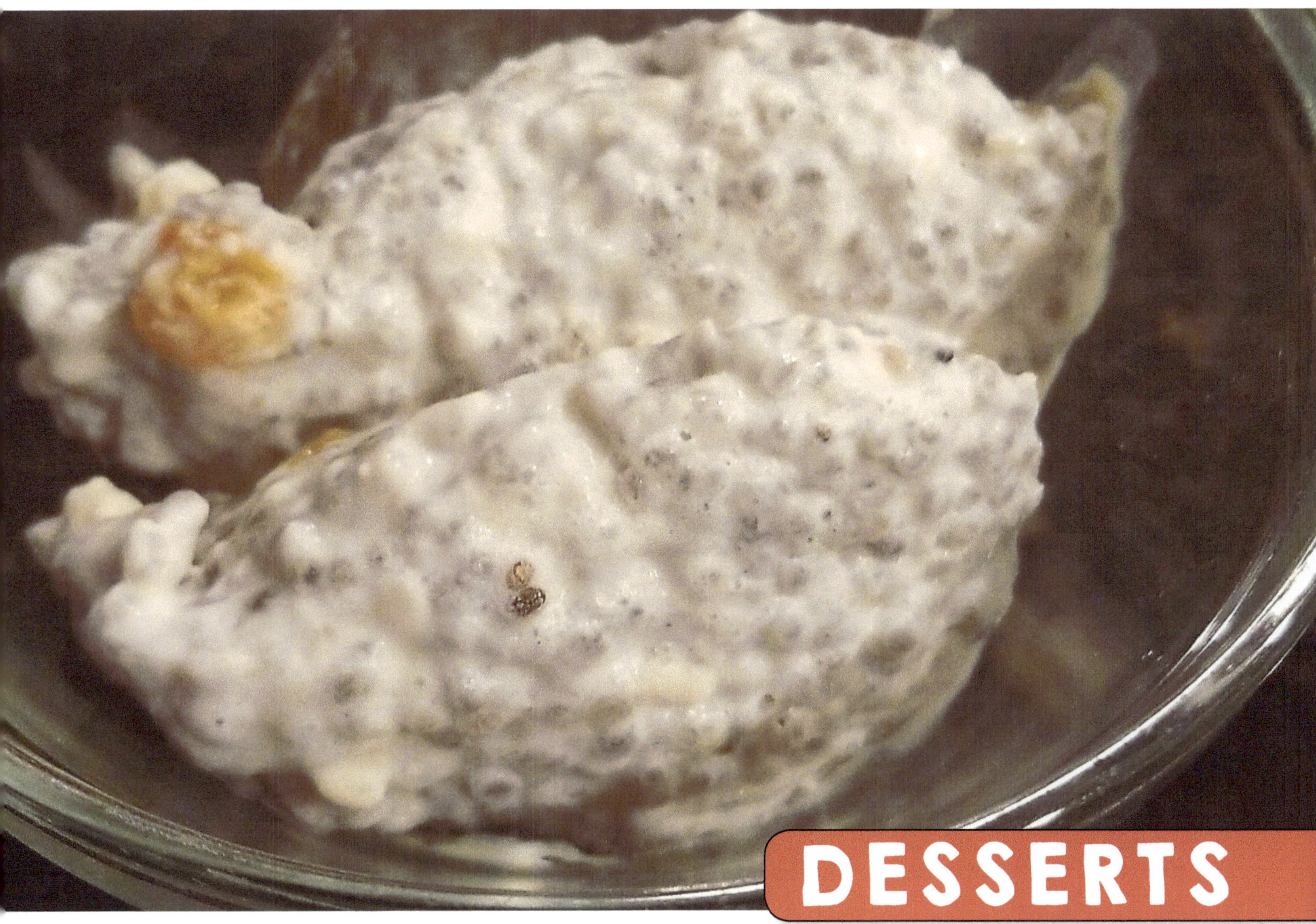

DESSERTS

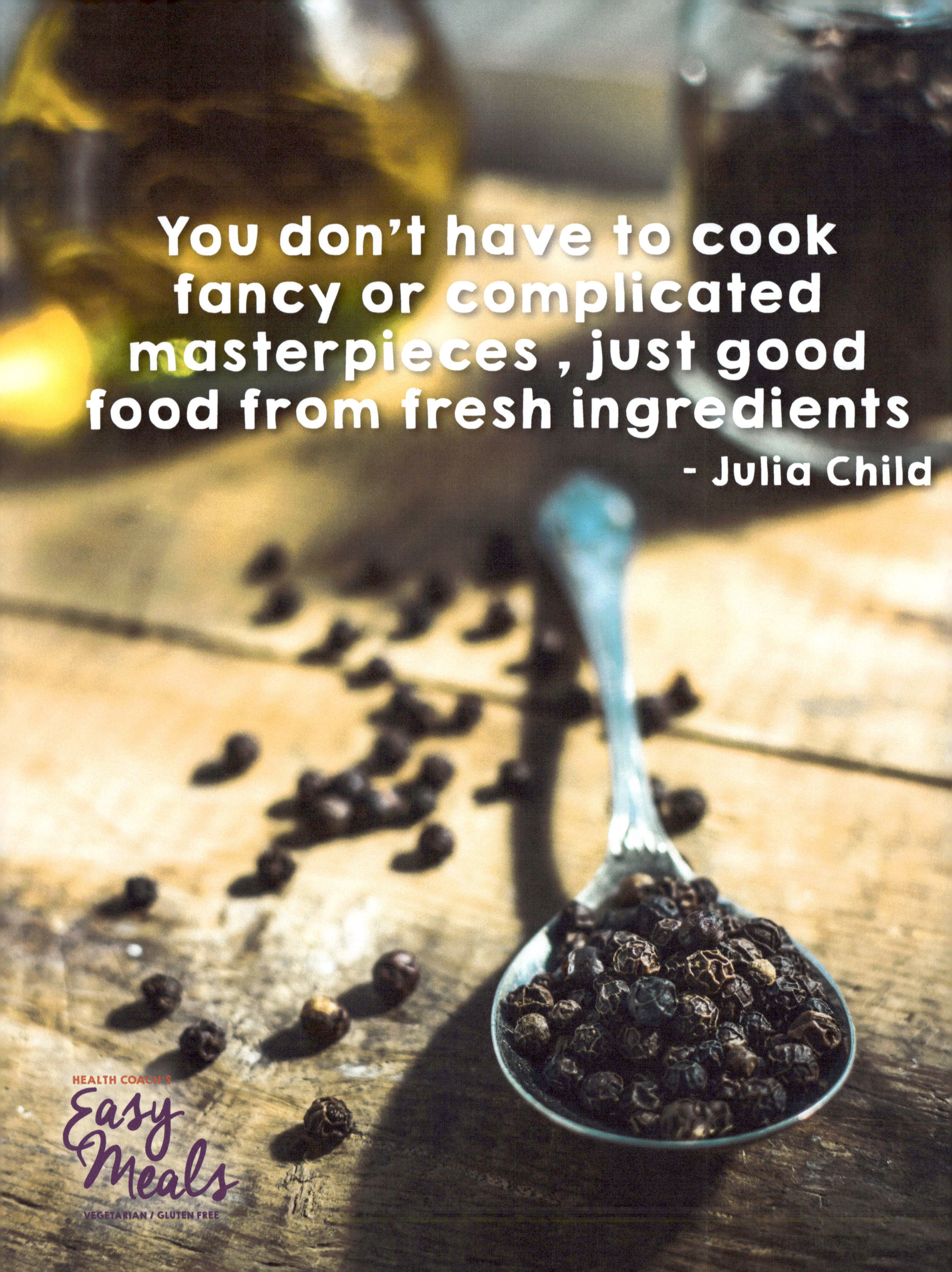
You don't have to cook fancy or complicated masterpieces , just good food from fresh ingredients
- Julia Child
HEALTH COACH'S
Easy Meals
VEGETARIAN / GLUTEN FREE

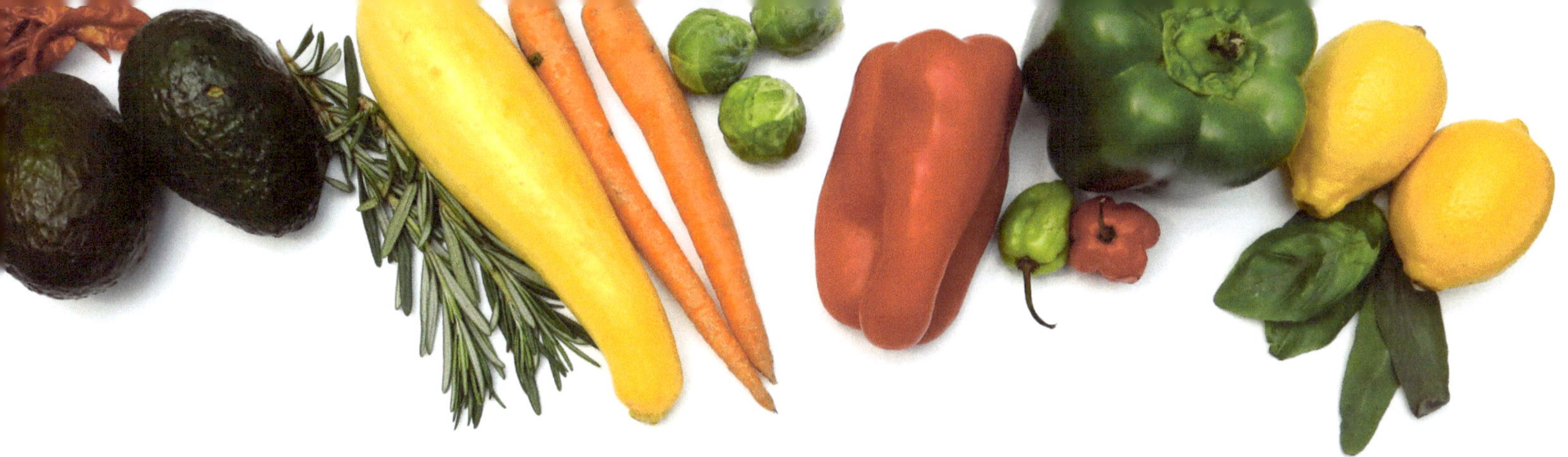

CONDIMENTS

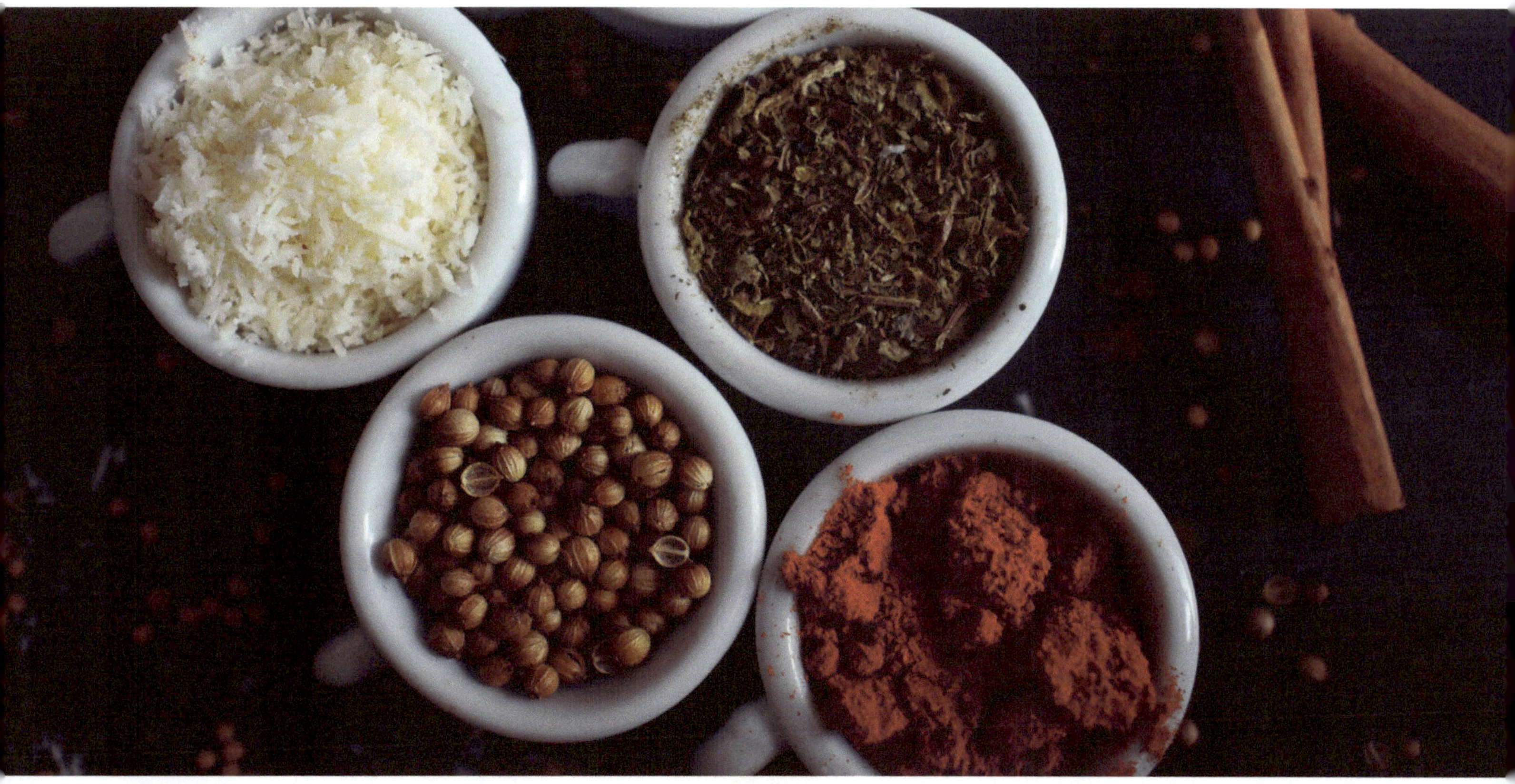

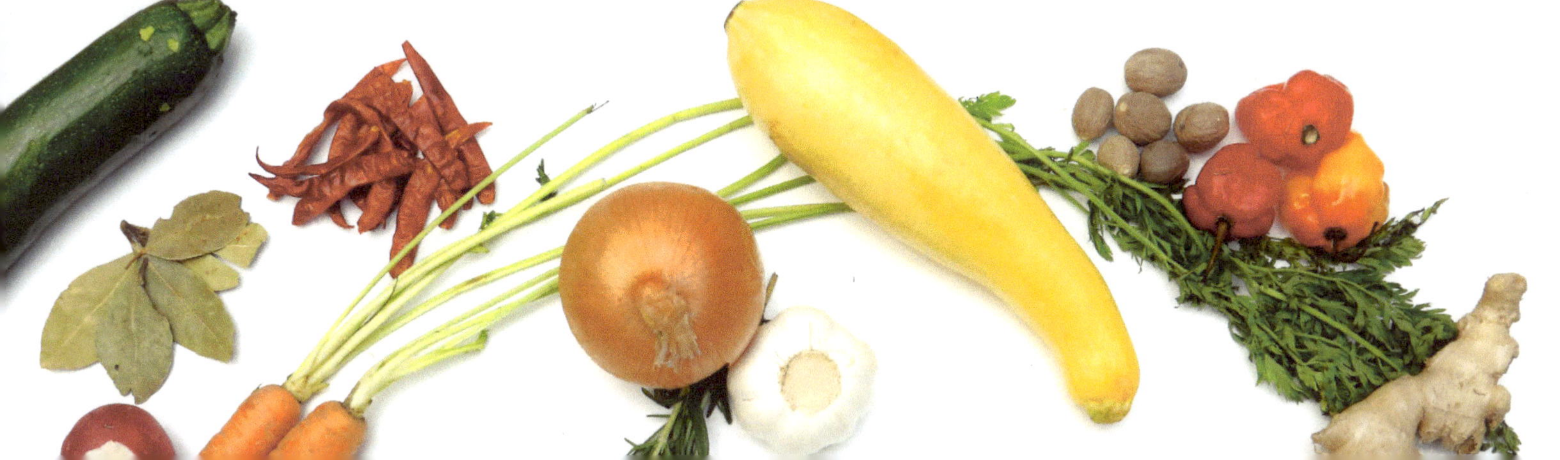

Green Mint Turmeric Chutney

INGREDIENTS

- 2 cups fresh mint leaves
- 1 medium size tomato
- 2 inch fresh ginger root
- 2 inch fresh turmeric root
- Salt and mango powder

DIRECTIONS

- Blend all the ingredients in blender for thick chutney.
- Keep refrigerated
- Serve as a dipping sauce or sandwich spread

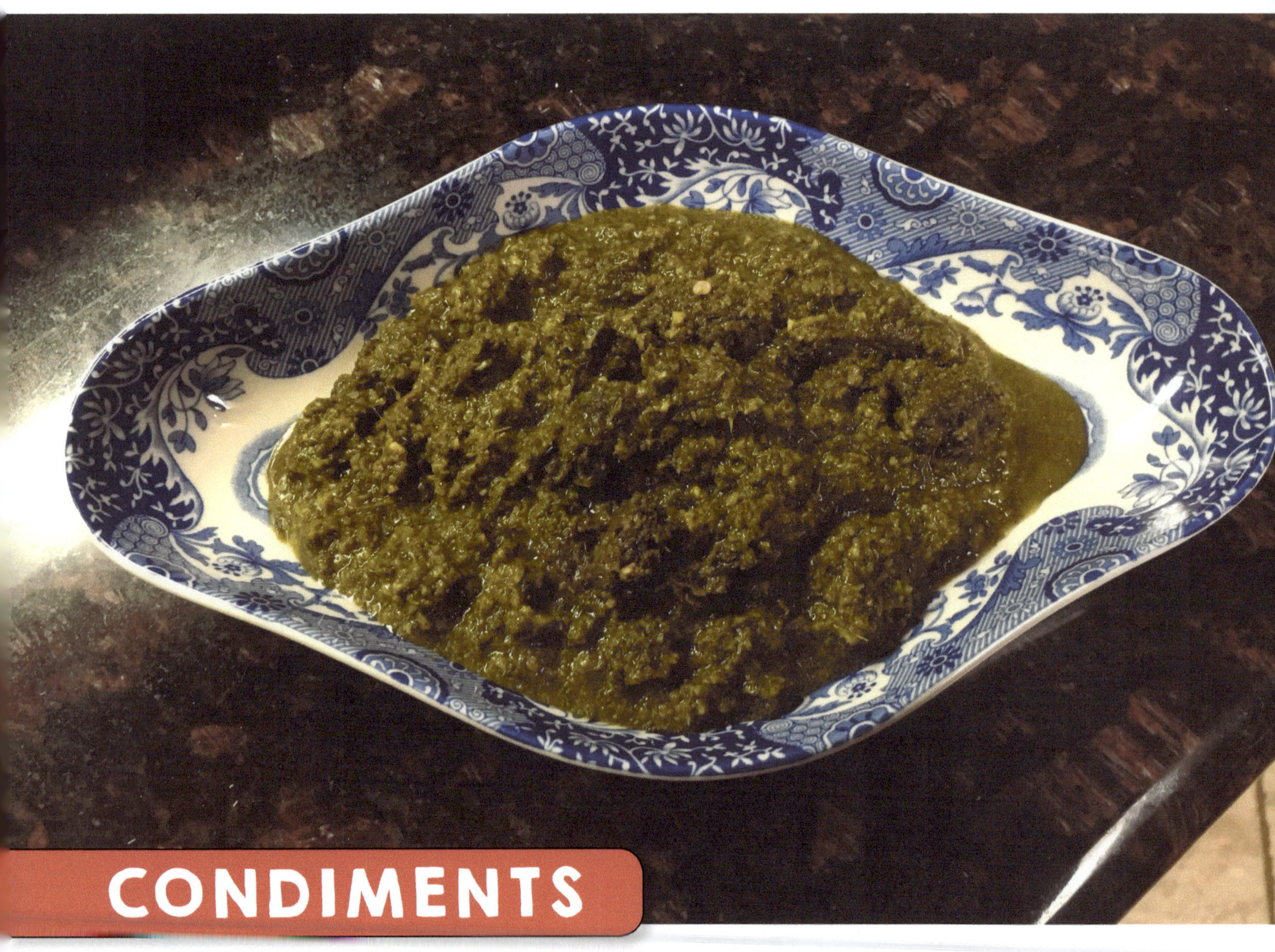

Coconut Chutney

INGREDIENTS

- ½ cup coconut cream
- a large handful of coriander (cilantro), roughly chopped
- 3 tbsp desiccated coconut (unsweetened)
- 1 habanero chilli, green chili or jalapeno chili roughly chopped
- 3 tsp lemon juice
- a pinch each of salt and freshly ground black pepper

DIRECTIONS

- Place the ingredients in a blender. Blend until smooth
- Place in a small covered bowl. Refrigerate until required.

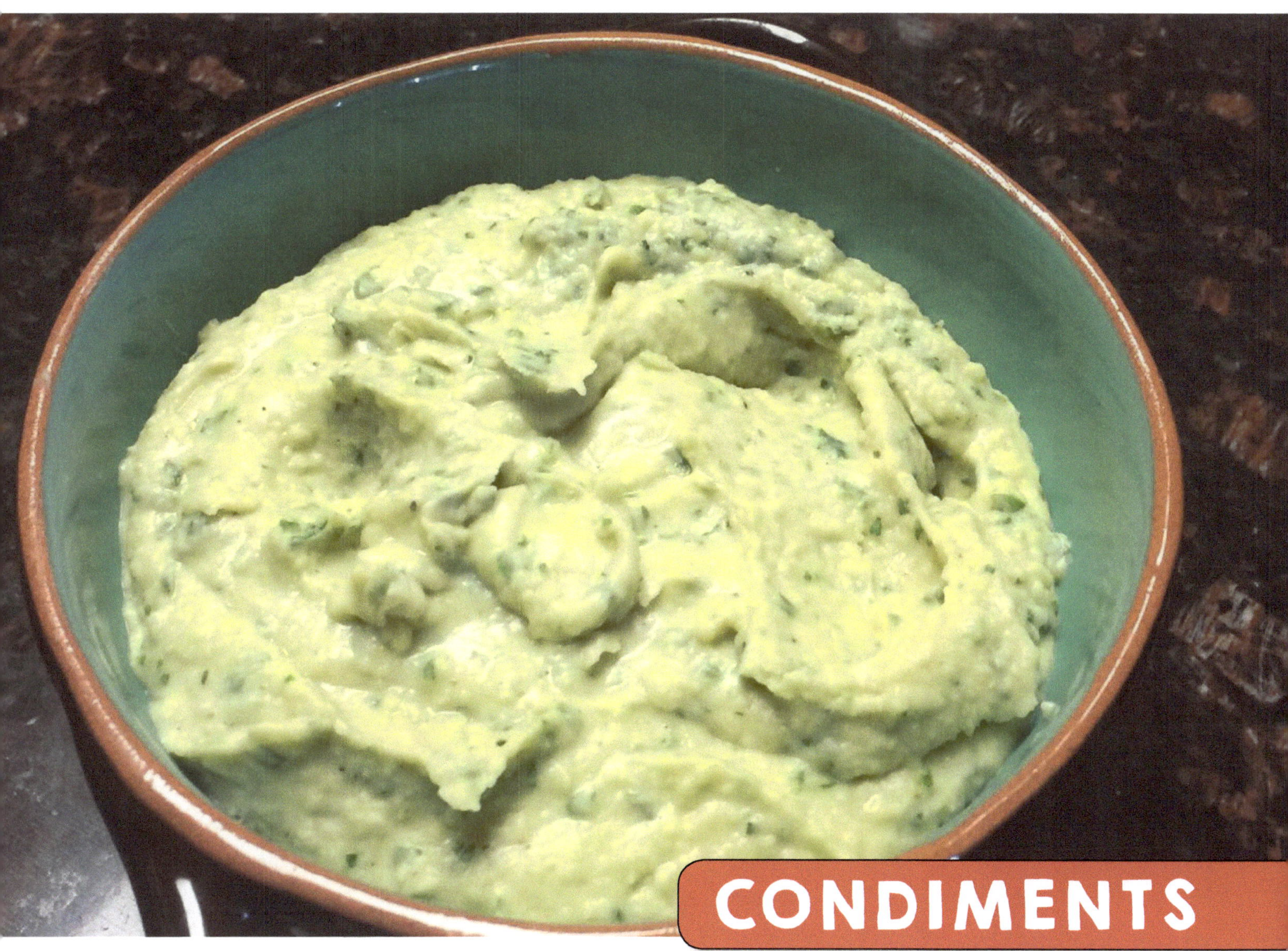

Mango Salsa

INGREDIENTS

- 1 Ripe mango, (large, cut into chunks
- 1/2 cup Tomatoes (diced)
- 1/2 cup Onion (diced)
- 1/2 cup Fresh cilantro (roughly chopped)
- 2 tbsp Juice from 2 limes
- Sea salt and fresh ground pepper (to taste)

DIRECTIONS

1. Mix diced mango, tomatoes, onion, and fresh cilantro together in a medium bowl.
2. Juice limes over diced salsa.
3. Add sea salt and pepper to taste.
4. Mix well, serve, and enjoy!

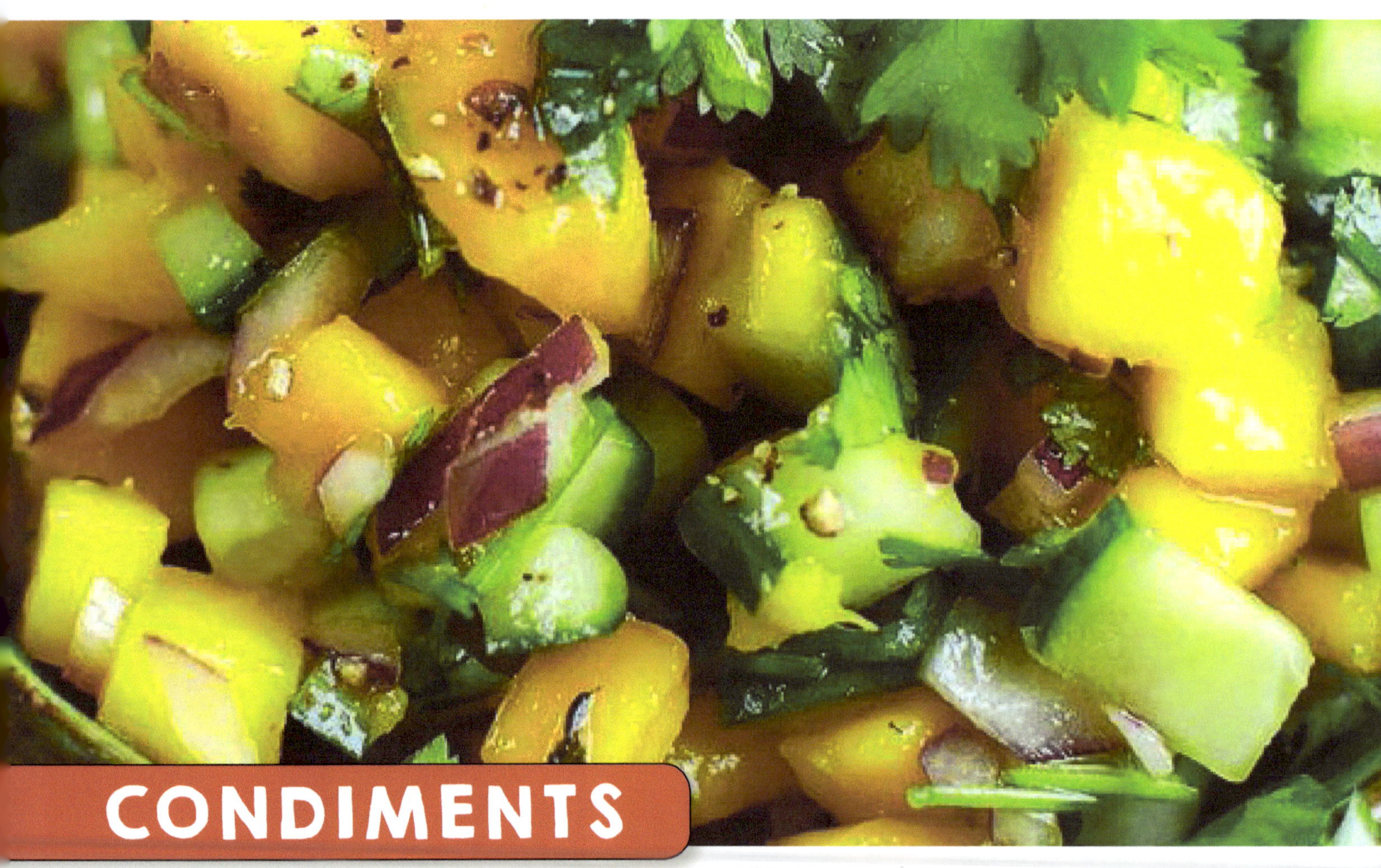

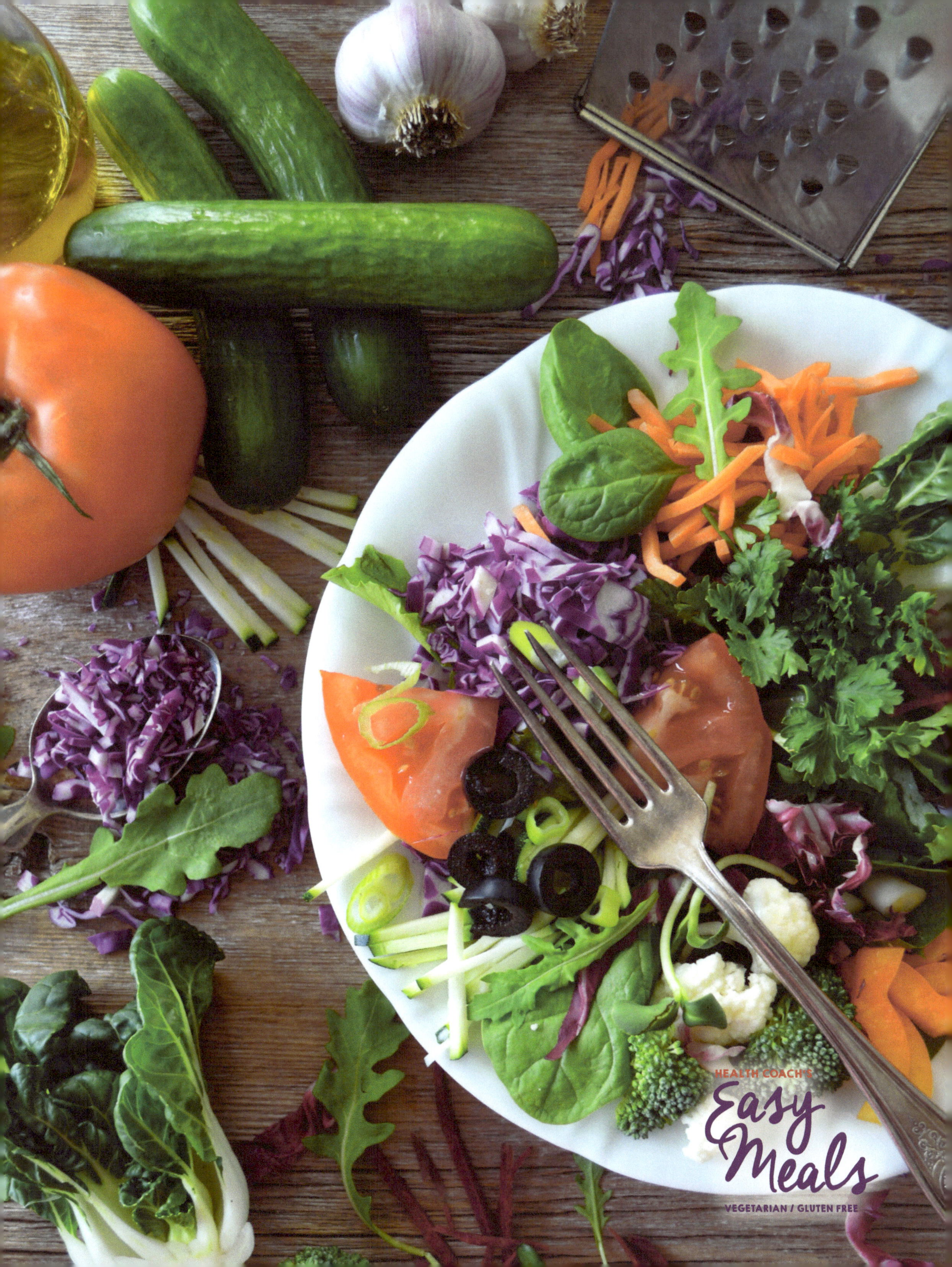

HEALTH COACH'S
Easy Meals
VEGETARIAN / GLUTEN FREE

CLEAN
UNPROCESSED
GLUTEN FREE
NUTRITIOUS
MACRONUTRIENTS
LEAN
VITAMINS
MINERALS
MICRONUTRIENTS
HEART HEALTHY
OMEGA 3
FIGURE FRIENDLY

www.ingramcontent.com/pod-product-compliance
Lightning Source LLC
Chambersburg PA
CBHW040141240726

48664CB00002B/559